# A Looming Shadow: The Threat of Drug-Resistant TB in South Africa

Catherine

First Printing, 2024

# TABLE OF CONTENTS

# CHAPTER ONE

# 1. Introduction

This chapter provides the key drug-resistant tuberculosis definitions used throughout the study and describes the rationale and background of this doctoral research project. This is followed by a general book overview including specific aims, hypothesis and objectives relevant to each chapter.

## 1.1 Key definitions

A broad range of terminology will be introduced and explained throughout the study cohort. However, it is imperative that key definitions are introduced at the beginning of this book (Table 1.1) [1].

**Table 1. 1** *Mycobacterium tuberculosis* classification of TB drugs according to definitions defined by the World

| ***Classification of anti-TB drugs based on resistance*** | ***Key definitions*** |
|---|---|
| Drug-resistant TB (DR-TB) | Resistance to any TB drug |
| Rifampicin-resistant TB (RR-TB) | Resistance to rifampicin with or without resistance to other TB drugs (includes RMR-TB, MDR-TB, pre-XDR-TB and XDR-TB) |
| Rifampicin mono-resistant TB (RMR-TB) | Resistance to rifampicin and susceptibility to isoniazid (regardless of susceptibility to other drugs) |
| Multi-drug resistant TB (MDR-TB) | Resistance to both rifampicin and isoniazid |
| Pre-extensively drug resistant TB (pre-XDR-TB) | MDR-TB with resistance to a fluoroquinolone OR a second-line injectable drug, but not both |
| Extensively-drug resistant TB (XDR-TB) | MDR-TB with resistance to a fluoroquinolone AND to at least one of the second-line injectable TB drugs |

**Note**: In the study cohort, MDR-TB comprised of both pre-XDR and XDR-TB

## 1.2 Background and Rationale

Drug-resistant TB (DR-TB) is a major concern worldwide, especially in South Africa. The burden of rifampicin-resistant TB (RR-TB) is becoming more apparent on a global scale [2]. There are a range of factors that likely contribute to a high burden of DR-TB worldwide. These factors may include HIV infection and its relation to active TB disease, as well as increased resistance of *Mycobacterium tuberculosis (M.tb)* to first line TB drugs [2]. In 2015, the World Health Organization (WHO) began using the term MDR/RR-TB, including all RR-TB (MDR- and RMR-TB) [3]. According to the WHO global TB report of 2019, there were an estimated 484 000 MDR/RR-TB cases globally in 2018, a number that has slightly declined compared to the 2017 global MDR/RR-TB case estimate (558 000) [2]. In South

Africa, 14 352 individuals were diagnosed with MDR/RR-TB in 2018, with an estimated incidence of 19/100 000/year [2].

The percentage of RMR-TB among all RR-TB varies dramatically across different settings globally, and constituted an estimated 22% and 38% globally and within South Africa, respectively, during 2018 (Figure 1.1) [2]. The WHO has also identified 30 high burden DR-TB countries, of which eight are African countries. Notably, some African and Central Asian countries had high estimates of RMR-TB in 2018; nearly as high as the estimated MDR-TB burden in those countries (Figure 1.1). In addition, it seems as though particular countries with high and low HIV-TB epidemics both report an estimated high proportion of RMR-TB; yet the reason for these variations is unclear (Figure 1.1) [2].

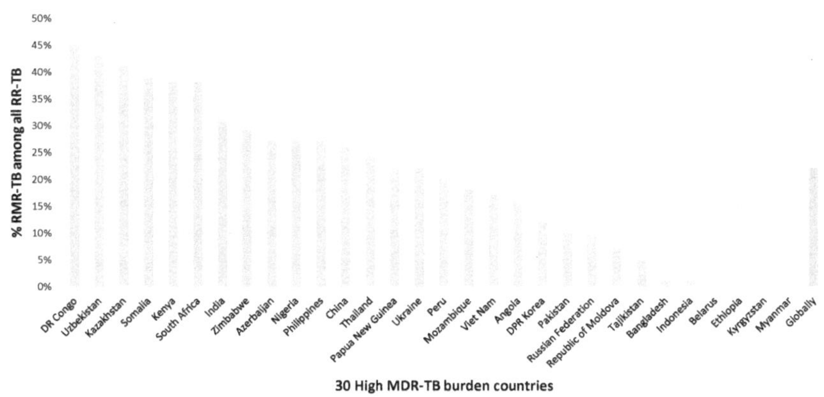


Adapted from: WHO global TB report 2019 [2]

**Figure 1. 1** Estimated percentage of RMR-TB among all RR-TB in 2018 for the 30 high MDR-TB burden countries globally

According to the South African national DR-TB survey results, there was a significant increase in the proportion of RMR-TB when compared to MDR-TB from the two surveys conducted during 2001-2002 and 2012-2014 (Figure 1.2). Moreover, throughout the nine provinces of South Africa, considerable variation in RMR-TB prevalence was found during the 2012-2014 DR-TB survey results (Figure 1.3).

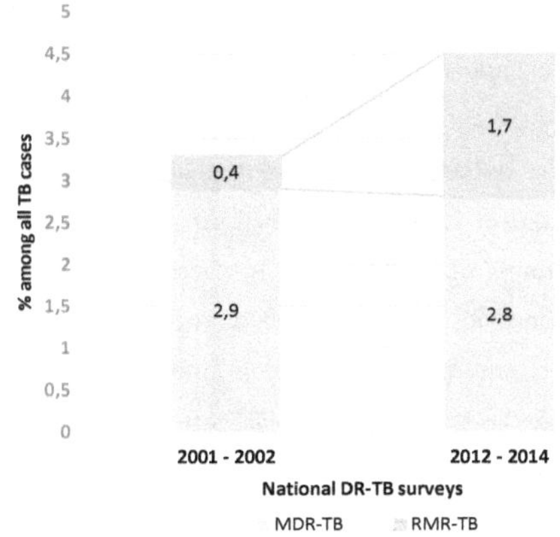


Adapted from: Ismail *et al.* [4]

**Figure 1. 2** Representation of RMR- and MDR-TB among all TB cases according to the South African drug-resistant TB survey results conducted during 2001-02 and 2012-14

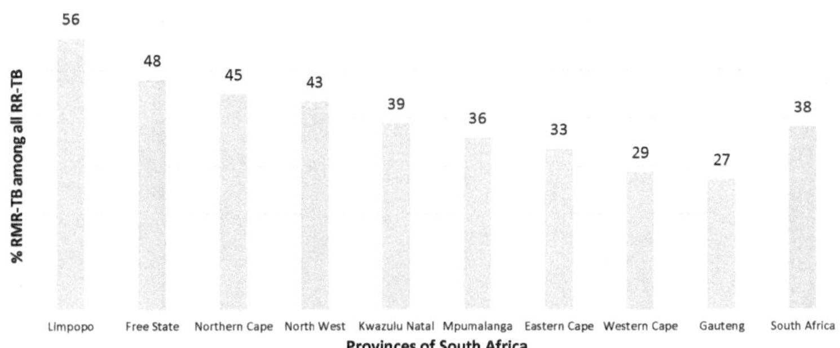


Adapted from: National Institute for Communicable Diseases 2016 [5]

**Figure 1. 3** Percentage of RMR-TB among all RR-TB across the 9 provinces in South Africa, according to the national DR-TB survey results conducted during 2012-14

Despite the above, research pertaining to RMR-TB is limited globally, especially in African countries. A recent study from Lesotho, identified a high proportion (33.7%) of RMR-TB among RR-TB between 2014-2016 [6]. Additional evidence of the high proportion of RMR-TB is similarly seen within particular provinces of South Africa [4, 7].

In this book, the study cohort is located in Khayelitsha within the Western Cape Province of South Africa; a high HIV, TB and DR-TB burden setting, providing a unique combination of high-quality routine data from diagnosed patients with RR-TB and a biobank of stored *M.tb* isolates over a long time. Together, these resources provide the potential to improve the understanding of DR-TB transmission and the impact of current control strategies. It has been shown through experimental and epidemiological data that the fitness of DR-TB strains is diverse and that the majority of the MDR-TB case burden may be transmitted rather than due to acquired resistance during patient treatment [8-10]. However, we do not know if the same theory applies for RMR-TB strains in the setting of Khayelitsha. Hence, this study intends to fill these knowledge gaps by investigating the emergence and spread of RMR-TB in Khayelitsha.

## 1.3 book overview

### 1.3.1 Aim of study

This study aims to improve the understanding of RR-TB transmission by describing the role of strain diversity and evolution of rifampicin resistance in *M.tb* strains, specifically in RMR- and MDR-TB strains from Khayelitsha, Cape Town, South Africa. This study is important as it will provide new insights that could assist in improving case detection and treatment, by providing knowledge of the acquisition and transmission of rifampicin resistance; and thereby contain the TB epidemic. There are several research objectives embedded within the overall aim of study (section 1.3.2), investigated in the subsequent chapters.

### 1.3.2 Overview of chapters

<u>Chapter 1</u>: **Introduction**

- Includes an overview of the study background; including study aims, hypothesis and objectives.

<u>Chapter 2</u>: **Literature review**

- Includes a literature review relevant to the book content.

<u>Chapter 3</u>: **Methodology**

- Describes the overall methods used within the relevant chapters throughout this study, and includes the study setting and design, ethical considerations and general overview of the workflow.

<u>Chapter 4</u>: **Temporal trends, transmission and risk factors associated with RMR-TB: a systematic review**

- A systematic review was conducted to assess published data from January 1990 until April 2019, on temporal trends, transmission and risk factors associated with RMR-TB.

<u>Chapter 5</u>: **Epidemiology of RMR-TB in Khayelitsha - The risk of RMR-TB relative to MDR-TB among RR-TB patients in Khayelitsha: impact of HIV infection during previous TB treatment**

- **Hypothesis:** HIV infection during first-line TB treatment is associated with a greater risk of subsequent RMR-TB relative to MDR-TB.
- **Objective a):** To describe the overall prevalence of RMR-TB among RR-TB patients diagnosed in Khayelitsha across 2008-2017 inclusive.
- **Objective b):** To assess the relative risk of RMR-TB versus MDR-TB among RR-TB patients diagnosed in Khayelitsha across 2013-2015 inclusive, by HIV and antiretroviral treatment (ART) status during prior TB treatment.

<u>Chapter 6</u>: **Mutations in *rpoB* and MICs found among RR-TB strains (Results)**

- **Hypothesis:** There is a difference in the distribution in rifampicin resistance associated mutations, as well as minimum inhibitory concentration (MIC) values among minimal and moderate confidence *rpoB* mutations between RMR-TB and MDR-TB.
- **Objective:** To compare the distribution of rifampicin resistance associated mutations, and to assess MIC values, among strains with particular rifampicin resistance associated *rpoB* mutations among RMR-TB and MDR-TB isolates, including minimal and moderate confidence *rpoB* mutations.

<u>Chapter 7</u>: **Mutations in *rpoB* and MICs found among RR-TB strains (Discussion)**

- Includes a discussion, describing literature in the context of the results obtained in Chapter 6.

<u>Chapter 8</u>: **Transmission cluster analysis (Results)**

- **Hypothesis:** RMR-TB strains are less fit and therefore less transmissible and/or less pathogenic.
- **Objective:** To assess if there is a difference in transmission success (based on strain clustering) among RMR-TB compared to that of MDR-TB strains.

<u>Chapter 9</u>: **Transmission cluster analysis (Discussion)**

- Includes a discussion, describing literature in the context of the results obtained in Chapter 8.

<u>Chapter 10</u>: **Key findings and general conclusions**

- Provides a summary of the key findings and concluding remarks of this doctoral research study and suggests prospective research developments.

# CHAPTER TWO

# 2. Literature review

## 2.1 Mechanisms of rifampicin resistance

In 1882, Robert Koch first identified the infectious agent *Mycobacterium tuberculosis* (*M.tb*), causing TB disease. In *M.tb,* drug resistance occurs through chromosomal mutations that often lead to a reduced growth rate termed a fitness cost [11, 12]. The fitness cost often corresponds to the position of resistance-conferring mutations and the number of such mutations in clinical isolates [13, 14]. Resistance-conferring mutations occur spontaneously at various rates for each *M.tb* drug (e.g rifampicin $2.25 \times 10^{-10}$, isoniazid $2.56 \times 10^{-8}$ mutation rate per bacterium per generation) [12]. Studies suggest that the fitness cost may be affected by epistasis [15, 16]; referred to as genetic interactions whereby the phenotypic effect of one mutation is established or modified by the presence of one or more other mutations in the same genome [17]. Thus, transmission success of drug resistance in TB is influenced by both epistasis and bacterial fitness; namely a function of growth rate, virulence and transmissibility [17].

Rifampicin (RIF), first introduced in 1972, is one of the most important first line TB drugs, and together with isoniazid (INH) forms the basis of the multidrug regimen for *M.tb* [18]. In most instances, RIF resistance (RIF R) is referred to as a surrogate marker for multi-drug resistant TB (MDR-TB) detection, as RIF R frequently occurs in strains that are also resistant to INH [19]. RIF acts to inhibit mycobacterial transcription by targeting DNA-dependent RNA polymerase, through binding to the ß-subunit of bacterial RNA polymerase that is encoded by the *rpoB* gene [19]. This leads to the inhibition of RNA transcription and protein synthesis in *M.tb* [18, 20].

In approximately 95% of RIF resistant *M.tb* strains, the primary mechanism conferring RIF R is due to mutations within the hot-spot region of the *rpoB* gene [19, 20]. This region is referred to as the rifampicin resistance determining region (RRDR) in cluster I, which not only occurs in *M.tb* but also in other organisms such as *Escherichia coli (E.coli)* [21, 22]. This RRDR region is 81 base pairs long; ranging from amino acids 507 to 533 when using the *E.coli* numbering system (Figure 2.1) [20, 22].

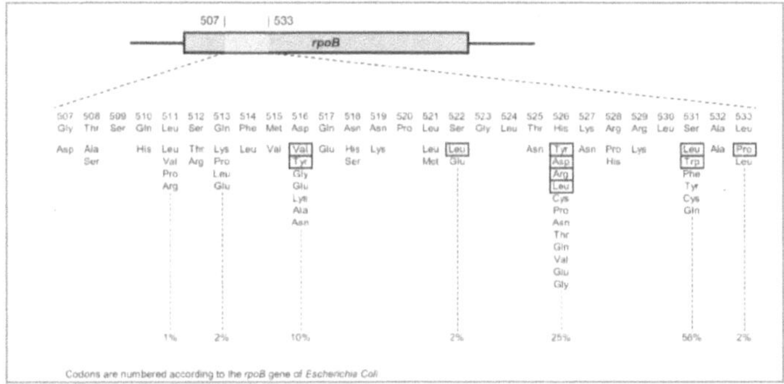


Pierre-Audigier *et al.* [22]

**Figure 2. 1** Missense mutations of the *rpoB* gene associated with rifampicin resistance in *M.tb*

It is important to note that the exact same mutations can be named differently depending on whether studies use the *E.coli* numbering system or the *M.tb* complex numbering system. These numbering systems may cause confusion as they differ depending on the location of the resistance conferring mutation [23]. In general, the number 81 is subtracted from a given codon in the *E.coli* numbering system (e.g. codon 531*)*, resulting in the *M.tb* complex numbering system (e.g. codon 450). However, codon 146 in the *E.coli* numbering system (located outside of the RRDR region), would require an additional number 24 to obtain the *M.tb* complex numbering system, namely codon 170 [23]. In this doctoral book, the *E.coli* gene nomenclature for naming *rpoB* mutations was used based on prior scientific resources [20, 23]. Additionally, reference was made to the *M.tb* complex numbering system later on in this book (Chapter six, Table 6.4).

The majority of RIF R *M.tb* strains may contain a single nucleotide polymorphism (SNP); which is a change in single nucleotide from the wild-type nucleotide at that position, mostly referred to as point mutations, insertions or deletions of a single base pair from a DNA sequence [19]. Furthermore, SNPs in the coding region are more frequently found as nonsynonymous SNPs (missense mutations), causing a change to a codon of an amino acid sequence protein. On the other hand, synonymous SNPs (silent mutations) do not cause structural changes to the amino acid sequence protein; thus, not interfering with its inhibition by RIF.

Mutations in the RRDR region that occur at codons 516, 526 and 531 are most commonly found among clinical isolates across most settings globally [24, 25]. High level phenotypic resistance to RIF is mainly found with amino acid alterations of codon 526 or 531, with minimum inhibitory concentrations greater than 32 µg/ml; as the standard critical concentration for RIF is ≤1 µg/ml (detailed explanation to follow in section 2.3.2). On the contrary, lower level phenotypic resistance to RIF is generally caused by mutations in codons 511, 516, 518, 522 and 533 [25]. Some of these low-level RIF R mutations (i.e. 511, 516, 533), are referred to as disputed *rpoB* mutations; causing discrepancies between genotypic and phenotypic drug susceptibility testing (pDST) [on the mycobacteria growth indicator tube (MGIT) liquid culture] [24, 26]. Studies have shown that disputed *rpoB* mutations occur in over 10% of RIF R isolates and can result in treatment failure in first line TB regimens [27]. Additionally, RIF R conferring mutations can be found outside of the hot-spot region of the *rpoB* gene, in low frequencies, namely in cluster N terminal (amino acids 146-148) and cluster II (amino acids 563-574 and 687); found in 5 to 10% RIF R strains [28, 29]. For instance, Sanchez-Padilla *et al.* [30] detected 30% (38/125 among MDR-TB strains) of *rpoB* I572F (I491F) *rpoB* mutation that was located outside of the RRDR region. This disputed mutation is often undetected by molecular (GeneXpert and line probe assay) and phenotypic (MGIT) tests, and has been reported to confer low-level RIF R [24, 26, 31]. Moreover, a population-level survey from seven countries detected only 1% (5/958 among all RR-TB strains) *rpoB* mutation I572F [32]. Three of the five mutations were found to be phenotypically susceptible, and two of the five mutations were phenotypically resistant [32]. Lastly, Ahmed *et al.* [33] found 8% of RIF resistant isolates in the *rpoB* N-terminal and cluster II mutations from Middle Eastern and South Asian TB patients.

## 2.2 Drug-resistant TB: Acquisition and transmission

There are two mechanisms by which patients may develop drug-resistant TB (DR-TB), namely: transmitted or primary drug resistance (often described as new TB cases); and acquired or secondary drug resistance (often described as prior TB treated cases). Transmitted drug resistance means that an individual has been directly infected with a DR-TB strain [34]. Acquired drug resistance is resistance that develops during TB therapy due to positive selection of drug-resistant mutants in the bacterial population. Hence, the global DR-TB epidemic is currently due to a combination of both transmission and acquisition [2]. The South African DR-TB epidemic also reports both transmission and acquisition demonstrated by several epidemiological and molecular studies [35-43].

There are many reasons that contribute to inadequate or ineffective TB treatment, that may cause acquired drug resistance. For instance, these include poor drug quality or poor treatment quality [44-46]; leading to the interruption of patients adherence to TB treatment (Figure 2.2) [38]. Even so, evidence shows that acquired drug resistance only occurs at the highest levels of poor adherence to treatment, and that pharmacokinetic variability is a more likely cause of resistance emergence [47]. Other reasons that may contibute to inadequate or ineffective TB treatment may include diagnostic delay or undiagnosed drug resistance, resulting in a higher bacterial burden; and drug malabsorption or drug to drug interactions leading to low serum levels (regardless of HIV status) (Figure 2.2) [48-50].

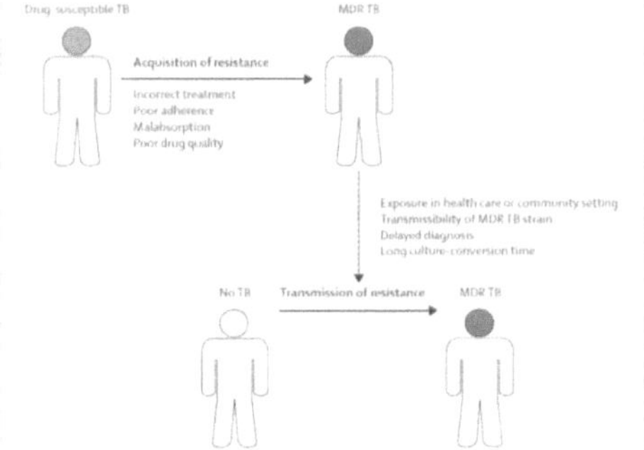


Ghandi *et al.* [38]

**Figure 2. 2** Mechanisms of drug-resistant TB

Just as for all TB (DR-TB and drug-susceptible TB [DS-TB]), environmental factors such as overcrowding, inadequate ventilation, poor infection control practices, and poor utilization of health care facilities may also contribute to the transmission of DR-TB. Similarly, patients with underlying immune suppression (for instance HIV infection, malnutrition, diabetes, silicosis, smoking, alcohol abuse, a wide range of systemic diseases and use of drugs with immunosuppressant properties) are also risk factors for the transmission and/or acquisition of DR-TB [34, 51-53]. Understanding the different *M.tb* strain population/s circulating in a specific region could help decipher *M.tb* transmission. For instance, the difference in phylogenetic lineages might recompense for fitness costs of acquired resistance, resulting in fast emergence of resistance in the course of treatment because of higher mutation rates or effective transmission of resistant strains [9, 54].

Moreover, recurrent TB episodes can be categorised as relapse (through inadequate TB treatment) or re-infection (through ongoing transmission with a newly infecting TB strain) [55, 56]. Genotypic studies performed on serial *M.tb* isolates found that re-infection with a new DR-TB strain may occur among previously TB treated patients [57-59]. Furthermore, within-host diversity can appear as mixed infections, for instance, a single infection with multiple distinct strains, i.e. DS-TB and DR-TB. Thus, mixed infections may result in undiagnosed drug resistance [60]. Furthermore, studies suggest that infection with more than one TB strain is frequently found in high HIV prevalence settings [59, 61, 62].

A systematic review by Hatherell *et al.* [63] outlines studies that describe the usefulness of whole genome sequencing (WGS) data in understanding transmission of TB. With that said, evidence now shows that transmission is playing an increasing role on the global burden of DR-TB [8, 38, 64-67]. For instance, Suen *et al.* [10] suggested that the cause of MDR-TB will shift from acquisition of resistance during treatment to direct person-to-person transmission of MDR-TB strains in high TB burden settings. Kendall *et al.* [8] described data on a dynamic transmission model, providing data from six countries from various settings, and estimated that most incident MDR-TB from the majority of high MDR-TB burden settings occurs as a result of transmission rather than treatment-related acquisition of resistance. Recently, Dadu *et al.* [68] showed that newly notified TB cases in eastern Europe and central Asia were either increasing (in eight countries) or remained stable (in seven countries) among DR-TB strains, specifically among MDR/RR-TB, when compared to DS-TB strains. Furthermore, only two of the 17 countries reported a decrease in DR-TB, demonstrating that the DR-TB epidemic is mostly driven by transmission, rather than acquired drug resistance in those areas. Moreover, China, Russia and central Asia, illustrated closely related and highly transmissible DR-TB strains by means of WGS [69, 70].

Evidence suggests that transmission of DR-TB among patients (with or without HIV-TB co-infection) may occur within hospital settings [71, 72], between household contacts [73-75], and within community settings such as shops, bars and restaurants (Figure 2.3) [67, 76, 77]. Furthermore, data from a Cape Town township (571 residents), in the Western Cape province of South Africa suggests that public transport, workplaces and schools are well known areas for *M.tb* transmission [78]. In addition, transmission may occur in other areas such as mines and prisons [79, 80], with migration also adding onto the spread of DR-TB across borders [36].

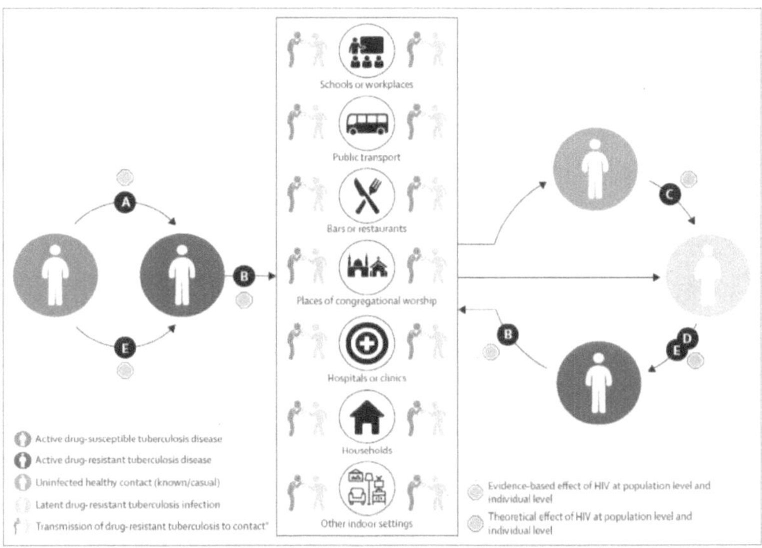


Khan *et al.* [67]

**Figure 2. 3** Diagrammatic representation of how HIV affects the transmission dynamics of drug-resistant tuberculosis

**(A)** Acquired drug resistance; **(B)** Transmitted drug resistance; **(C)** Establishment of DR-TB infection; **(D)** Progression from recently acquired or latent infection to active disease; **(E)** Reinfection or superinfection with DR-TB; Contact can either be uninfected, healthy, with a latent infection or an active disease [drug-susceptible or drug-resistant TB]

## 2.3 Diagnosis of drug-resistant TB

Historically, the diagnosis of *M.tb* relied on microscopy through examination of a stained sputum smear containing acid fast bacilli (referred to as a sputum smear positive result). However, culture is more sensitive for *M.tb* detection than microscopy. Drug susceptibility testing (DST) to a range of first- and second-line drugs is required for the successful diagnosis and treatment of *M.tb*, specifically DR-TB [38]. The diagnosis of DR-TB is either assessed genotypically with rapid molecular tests (identifying resistance conferring mutations) or phenotypically with culture-based methods, ideally in biosafety level 3 laboratories (liquid or solid culture growth in the presence of a *M.tb* drug) [38, 81]. However, culture-based pDST is labour intensive and does not provide rapid results (longer incubation period). Another disadvantage of pDST is the lack of reproducibility and accuracy, specifically for drugs like pyrazinamide [82]. For these reasons, molecular tests are increasingly used for the detection of *M.tb* and DR-TB worldwide [83].

### 2.3.1 Genotypic drug susceptibility testing

Rapid molecular/genotypic tests identify variants in the RRDR region of the *rpoB* gene for detection of rifampicin-resistant TB (RR-TB). These molecular tests are increasingly used to effectively diagnose and treat RR-TB patients. In 2008, the World Health Organization (WHO) endorsed the GenoType MTBDR*plus* line probe assay (LPA) [Hain Lifescience, Nehren, Germany] for detection of DR-TB in high HIV and MDR-TB settings [83]. Subsequently, in 2010 and 2017, the WHO endorsed the GeneXpert MTB/RIF (Xpert) and GeneXpert MTB/RIF Ultra assays [Cepheid, Sunnyvale, USA], respectively [83]. Xpert rapidly detects *M.tb* and resistance to RIF, whereas LPA detects resistance to both RIF and INH [84, 85]. Both molecular methods have a short turnaround time, with Xpert (from *M.tb* in specimens) taking less than a day (estimated 2 to 4 hours) and the LPA (if done directly on smear positive specimens or on a cultured *M.tb* isolate), approximately 24 to 48 hours [84, 85]. In South Africa, the initial detection of RR-TB is with Xpert, followed by the LPA to assess for MDR-TB [86]. However, discordance may occur between the results of these two molecular tests. Similarly, van Rie *et al.* [87], observed a relatively high discordance (9.6%) among RR-TB between routinely diagnosed Xpert and LPA results during 2012-2013 within three provinces of South Africa (Eastern Cape, Free State and Gauteng). Possible reasons for discordance were either the presence of variants not included in mutant probes in the LPA test, heteroresistance, a false-positive according to molecular testing, a sample mix-up, or administrative errors [87].

Furthermore, the LPA may often underestimate resistance to INH. This is mainly due to a limited number of INH resistant mutations that are detected by the LPA. Therefore, as a result of limitations of molecular based diagnostic tests, the misreporting of MDR-TB as rifampicin mono-resistant TB (RMR-TB) is more likely. Data from all TB cases from 25 public health clinics in South Africa, observed 0.2% of RMR-TB cases before the introduction of the LPA and 1.8% of RMR-TB cases after the introduction of the LPA [88]. This suggests that the LPA over-diagnoses RMR-TB cases. In response, it was proposed by Coovadia *et al.* [89] that to avoid misclassification of RMR-TB detected by Xpert as MDR-TB, a culture based INH pDST should be performed on a second specimen. These guidelines are recommended by the WHO and the South African National Department of Health (SA NDoH). However, any discordance may lead to confusion to the clinicians decision of TB diagnosis as the impact of discordance on treatment outcomes is not that simple. This could lead to additional laboratory testing with delayed treatment initiation that is quite challenging to the clinical management of patients [87]. Thus, this may cause implications on the patients health due to overtreatment of TB drugs that may cause various side effects that varies between patients and different social contexts [90, 91]. As a result, potential strain on the increase expenditure within healthcare systems may occur as the number of people being treated for TB are multiplied [90, 92]. Furthermore, second-line TB drugs tend to be more expensive resulting in additional long-term patient follow-up commonly found among second-line TB treatment patients potenially resulting in poorer patient treatment outcomes. Lastly possible transmission of DR-TB strains within the community could manifest [90, 93].

### 2.3.2 Phenotypic drug susceptibility testing

Despite the fact that the WHO recommends Xpert testing for the initial diagnosis of screening RIF R in all patients in many settings, conventional microscopy and phenotypic culture-based DST is of utmost importance for diagnosing DR-TB together with monitoring the treatment progress of patients [81]. However, the turnaround time for either liquid or solid culture DST, could take weeks or months of incubation, due to the slow growth of *M.tb* [94, 95]. Nonetheless, pDST can detect DR-TB or DS-TB based on growth in the presence of a critical concentration (CC) of a TB drug. This CC is defined as the lowest drug concentration that inhibits ≥95% of wild-type strains of *M.tb* not previously exposed to the drug [96]. The minimum inhibitory concentration (MIC) is defined as the lowest drug concentration needed to prevent visible growth of more than 99% of the *M.tb* population in the presence of a drug [97]. The highest MIC within the wild-type MIC distribution is defined as the epidemiological cut-off (ECOFF). The MIC value of a drug concentration is interpreted as either susceptible (wild-type strains) or resistant (non-wild-type strains) [97].

Solid culture DST comprises agar or egg-based media, for instance Löwenstein-Jensen (LJ) media. This method depends on the CC of the drug and the number of resistant *M.tb* bacilli in a population [98]. A comparison [ratio] is made between the number of colony forming units that grows within the drug containing media (i.e. the number of resistant bacilli in the inoculum dilution); and the drug free media (i.e. the number of viable bacilli in the corresponding dilution) [98]. An isolate is reported as susceptible if the ratio is below the critical proportion (1%), and resistant if the ratio is above 1%. For the interpretation of solid culture DST, the control media should have a minimum of 20 countable colonies [98, 99]. Nonetheless, technical errors such as the incorrect preparation of inoculum size could potentially lead to contamination, false resistant or false susceptible results [98, 99].

On the other hand, liquid culture DST like the MGIT, contains 7ml modified Middlebrook 7H9 broth. The Bactec MGIT 960 system is used for primary isolation and DST of first and second-line TB drugs as recommended by the manufacturer from pure cultures on *M.tb* isolates [100]. The MGIT 960 system is used in conjunction with the EpiCenter software with the TB eXiST module. For quantitative DST using the MGIT 960, the software is designed with the following characteristics: automated recording of the readings, additional incubation time beyond the time to positivity of the drug-free control, minimization of the number of drug-free control tubes required, graphical representation of the growth unit (GU) value increase and storage of data, and easy handling and documentation [101].

By using molecular assays, many studies have also highlighted discrepancies between conventional phenotypic and genotypic DST results for various first and second-line TB drugs [102]. The following three key points indicate the importance of understanding the individual mutations contribution to the drug-resistance phenotype in *M.tb*; i) different mutations of the same genomic region may cause different MIC values; ii) the same mutations can cause variable levels of resistance to different members of the same drug class; iii) the same mutations can cause different MIC levels in different strains, indicating a role for genetic background of the isolate. For instance, some mutations in the *rpoB* gene can lead to different levels of resistance to RIF and some mutations require specific genetic background for driving the development of resistance. Also, some *rpoB* mutations showed different MIC values and susceptibility results among different testing methods [102].

## 2.4 Molecular epidemiology of TB

Traditionally, the most commonly used genotyping methods for investigating *M.tb* epidemiology are IS*6110* restriction fragment length polymorphism (RFLP), spoligotyping and mycobacterial interspersed repetitive units of variable-number tandem repeats (MIRU-VNTR). IS*6110* is an insertion sequence in the *M.tb* genome widely used as a genetic marker with IS*6110* RFLP; namely the first gold standard method used for *M.tb* genotyping [103, 104]. This genotyping method has successfully been used to define transmission, differentiate relapse from re-infection, and detect laboratory cross contamination [105, 106]. Polymerase chain reaction (PCR) based techniques such as spoligotyping, are used to determine the presence or absence of 43 interspersed spacer sequences in the direct repeat region within *M.tb* strains [107]. The international spoligotyping database groups strains into different clades or families based on similarity in a spoligotyping pattern [108]. Hence, this technique was found to have less discriminatory power than IS*6110* RFLP [109]; whereas MIRU-VNTR has a higher discriminatory power than IS*6110* RFLP [103]. MIRU-VNTR is based on PCR amplification using a standardised set of 12 or 24 loci with the ability to determine mixed subpopulations from sputum specimens [110]. However, implementation of MIRU-VNTR in Europe was found to be technically complex with poor reproducibility, also showing insufficient discriminatory power [111, 112]. Overall, the above genotyping methods are time consuming, labour intensive, technically demanding, and require large amounts of good quality DNA from *M.tb* isolates [107].

Genomic deletions, namely large sequence polymorphisms (LSPs) or regions of differences (RDs) are generally used as markers to classify groups of *M.tb* strains into phylogenetic lineages [113-117] and sublineages [118, 119]. However, LSPs cannot differentiate between closely related strains; i.e. within a transmission chain or outbreak. Recently though, next generation sequencing (NGS) has been used to determine a nucleotide sequence of amplified DNA at specific loci of interest to give insight into the genomic evolution of *M.tb* [107]. Notably, whole genome sequencing (WGS) provides insight across the whole genome of *M.tb* in a given sample, revealing all mutation types and providing the best discriminatory power to differentiate between closely related strains. Notably, WGS analysis pipelines generally exclude ~10% of the genome as inaccurate mapping in various regions leads to false variant calls (PE and PPE gene families, repetitive genes, mobile genetic elements) [120]. Therefore the application of different criteria (read depth, base quality and strand bias) is used to filter out false positive variants [120]. Nonetheless, both sequencing methods have potential benefits to rapidly diagnose DR-TB in various clinical reference laboratory settings worldwide, by providing detailed information for multiple gene regions (namely NGS) or whole genomes of interest (namely WGS) [121]. However, there are still concerns regarding the implementation of NGS/WGS technologies for the diagnosis of DR-TB, especially in low- and middle-income countries. Some of these concerns include higher costs, technical training, and additional skills requirements for staff utilizing these technologies, the merging of these technologies into the existing laboratory workflow, and guidance given from experts on the management and clinical interpretation of sequencing data received [83].

Nevertheless, WGS has been used in various studies to investigate the evolution of DR-TB; with different approaches being used to differentiate drug susceptible and drug resistant clinical strains of TB. These include further investigation of phylogeny [122], molecular epidemiology [123-125] and mutation frequency analyses (i.e. transmission analyses) [126]. All these studies found novel bacterial genes and intergenic regions whose function may be ancillary to drug-resistance mutations. Thus, WGS offers more opportunities with considerably more information and accuracy when compared to traditional genotyping methods; both in research and public health sectors [127-129]. So far, the implementation of WGS in TB reference laboratories worldwide has proved to be a more time- and cost-effective technique compared to traditional diagnostic methods [130, 131].

For implementation of NGS/WGS in research or diagnostics, the workflow would include DNA extraction from a cultured *M.tb* specimen, library preparation, sequencing and data analysis. More recently though, studies show that WGS can be performed directly from sputum samples [132].

However, a high level of DNA contamination was found in extracted *M.tb* DNA from sputum samples when WGS was performed on the MiSeq (Illumini San Diego, CA) [133]. Another study performed WGS (MiSeq) by using a targeted enrichment approach (with oligonucleotide baits) to capture the DNA. Despite good depth of coverage (>20x) and genome coverage (>98%), the associated costs were not suitable for implementation thereof, particularly in low- and middle-income countries [134]. Hence, WGS performed directly from sputum samples will require further optimization [83]. Importantly, extracted DNA should be of high quality and quantity in order to generate high quality sequencing data for downstream NGS/WGS analysis [135].

Walker *et al.* [136] provides an overview of an in-house bioinformatics pipeline and its application to *M.tb* sequencing. Generally, WGS bioinformatics pipelines are either developed in-house based on open source modules; or are open-sourced and commercially available. Moreover, there are currently four *M.tb* web servers (CASTB, PhyResSE providing information directly to ReSeqTB, TB profiler and GenTB), and two software solutions (KvarQ and Mykrobe PredictorTB) that have been designed to facilitate the interpretation and analysis of *M.tb* drug resistance from genomic data [137-141].

## 2.5 Whole genome sequencing based TB diagnostics

TB profiler by Coll *et al.* [142], presented accuracy data comparing *in silico* whole genome analysis for resistance to 11 anti-TB drugs to conventional DST. Furthermore, they compared their curated mutation database to two others (*TBDReaMDB* and *MUBII-TB-DB*), as well as those used in three commercial molecular tests, namely i) the Xpert MTB/RIF (Cepheid, Inc., Sunnyvale, CA, USA) targeting the *rpoB* gene for RIF R ii) the LPA MTBDRplus (Hain Life Science, Germany) targeting *rpoB, katG* and *inhA* genes for resistance to RIF and INH, and iii) the LPA MTBDRsl (Hain Life Science, Germany) targeting *gyrA, rrs* and *embB* for resistance to fluoroquinolones, aminoglycocides and ethambutol, respectively. The library has been shown to be more accurate than alternative mutation databases and current commercial molecular tests. Moreover, Macedo *et al.* [143] evaluated four major online platforms (TB Profiler, PhyResSE, Mykrobe Predictor and TGS-TB) for the rapid prediction of resistance in a TB laboratory. TB profiler also proved to perform the best with regards to robustness (sensitivity, specificity, PPV and NPV above 95%), followed by TGS-TB (all parameters above 90%). Furthermore, the newer version of TB profiler by Phelan *et al.* [141], demonstrated superior predictive performance across first and second-line drugs when compared to other platforms (e.g. Mykrobe Predictor, the CRyPTIC library).

Authors suggest the technological transition where WGS-based bioinformatics platforms could eventually replace pDST for TB in future [144, 145]. Importantly, factors such as cost effectiveness, maintenance support, ease of use, analysis speed, accuracy (in association with phenotypic results), for NGS/WGS platforms should first be taken into consideration. Furthermore, the analysis of sequencing data is quite complex and will require healthcare workers to be trained on guidelines to determine the clinical relevance of genomic mutations detected by NGS/WGS technologies [146]. Thus, Miotto and colleagues [147], extracted data to conduct a comprehensive systematic review; developing a standardised analytical approach for sequencing and pDST data for a selection of *M.tb* drugs (INH, RIF, pyrazinamide, fluoroquinolones and second-line injectables) and their corresponding resistance genes. Collectively, the data were used to calculate the association of mutations with phenotypic drug resistance by obtaining likelihood ratios (LR) and odds ratios (OR) (Table 2.1). Furthermore, *M.tb* mutations were graded into confidence categories for the association between drug resistance associated mutations and phenotypic (liquid and solid media) drug resistance; by using an expert, consensus-driven approach [148-150]. A list of confidence-graded mutations were considered as conferring resistance to *M.tb* drugs associated with phenotypic drug resistance (determined by the best confidence values); and classified into high, moderate, minimal or indeterminate (not associated with resistance) confidence categories (Table 2.1; Table 2.2). The confidence graded list of first and second-line TB mutations would certainly be of great value for the interpretation of future pilot studies for WGS-based diagnostics in order to assist clinicians with the future possibility of individualised TB treatment regimens; containing the least toxic, most effective TB drug combinations for patients [147].

**Table 2. 1** Representation of the proposed confidence levels for grading mutations associated with phenotypic drug resistance

| | Symbol | LR⁺ and OR | |
|---|---|---|---|
| | | p-value | value |
| **High (Hi) confidence for association with resistance**<br>Strong association of the mutation with phenotypic drug resistance; sufficient evidence that the mutation confers or is strongly associated with drug resistance | # • | <0.05 | >10 |
| **Moderate (Mo) confidence for association with resistance**<br>Moderate association of the mutation with phenotypic drug resistance; additional data desirable for improved evidence that the mutation confers or is strongly associated with drug resistance | # | <0.05 | 5< ... ≤10 |
| **Minimal (Mi) confidence for association with resistance**<br>Weak association of the mutation with phenotypic drug resistance; inconclusive evidence that the mutation confers or is strongly associated with drug resistance. Substantial additional data required | # • | <0.05 | 1< ... ≤5 |
| **No association with resistance**<br>No evidence of association between the mutation and drug resistance | # • | <0.05 | <1 |
| **Indeterminate**<br>No statistically significant threshold reached; additional data required | Indeter | ≥0.05 | |

Miotto *et al.* [147]

**Note:** Thresholds are applied to likelihood ratios and odds ratios to grade the association of mutations with phenotypic drug resistance. **Abbreviations:** LR⁺ (positive likelihood ratio); OR (odds ratio). **Terminology:** "Additional data" = a requirement for more phenotypically drug resistant and susceptible isolates needed to be tested with a particular mutation; and/or a better understanding of drug resistance mechanisms (i.e. research regarding epistasis, interactions between drug-resistance conferring mutations, lineage-specific genetic factors, compensatory mutations, or synergistic factors when not only one mutation is required to confer drug resistance)

**Table 2. 2** A confidence-graded *rpoB* mutation list with phenotypic drug resistance as determined by best confidence levels for rifampicin only

| Drug (phenotypic testing) | Gene | High-confidence mutations | Moderate-confidence mutations | Minimal-confidence mutations |
|---|---|---|---|---|
| First-line | | | | |
| Rifampicin (R) | *rpoB* | F505V+D516Y, S512T, Q513H+L533P, Q513-F514ins, **Q513K**, **Q513L**, **Q513P**, **F514dupl**, M515I+D516Y, **D516A**, **D516F**, **D516G**, D516G+L533P, D516ins, D516N, **D516V**, Del N518, **S522Q**, **H526C**, **H526D**, H526F, **H526G**, **H526L**, **H526R**, **H526Y** **S531F**, **S531L**, S531Q, **S531W**, S531Y, D626E | **D516Y**, **S522L**, H526P, **L533P** | **L511P**, **H526N**, **I572F** |

Miotto *et al.* [147]

**Note**: Details for the remaining first and second-line TB drugs are also listed in the article. Standard text in the table illustrates associations based on nominal p-values (putative); Bold text illustrates associations based on corrected p-values

## 2.6 Whole genome sequencing and TB strain diversity

The use of WGS has provided valuable insights into the epidemiology of *M.tb* and DR-TB, even in low-income settings such as South Africa, Nigeria, Malawi, Greenland and Belarus [35, 151-153]. Additionally, WGS also allows differentiation between relapse and reinfection, measurement of within-host diversity, potential impact on transmission, and identifying primary versus acquired drug resistance in various settings [154] . Relapse suggests inadequate treatment where the patient had treatment but is still infected and active disease re-emerges. Reinfection implies ongoing transmission requiring public health action, suggesting a lack of immunity to the newly infecting strain or high intensity of exposure. Furthermore, within-host diversity may arise from mixed infections (a single infection even with multiple distinct strains or repeated infection events with distinct strains (e.g. superinfection) or microevolution (within-host evolution). Overall, studies with WGS have reported several findings that are important for understanding transmission of TB [155]. Diversity plays a significant role in transmission and a large number of SNPs can be found between cross-sectional samples from a patient. A combination of WGS data, epidemiological data and clinical history is therefore important to strengthen investigations of *M.tb* transmission [63].

Evidence shows that the *M.tb* genomic mutation (or transmission rate) may vary from an estimated 0.3 to 1.1 SNPs per genome per year [156-158], or by 0.003 SNPs per day [151]. In the past, research has shown that genetic distances between strains within a SNP distance of 0-5, confirmed epidemiological links between strains isolated from patients [63, 156, 157, 159, 160]. Thus, according to epidemiological observations and the genomic mutation rate, a SNP threshold of ≤5 indicated recent transmission [156, 161], whereas strains with more than 12 SNPs apart were not considered to be directly transmitted between patients. For this reason, the most frequently used SNP threshold of 12 is commonly used for inferring possible transmission between TB cases [156, 162]. Additionally, a systematic review published in 2016, provided confirmation of this from 12 studies [163]. Despite this, the *M.tb* genomic mutation rate may vary across different settings (i.e. high DR-TB and HIV prevalence settings) [151].

Another factor that could potentially increase the transmission of *M.tb* strains is phylogenetic lineages. The *M.tb* complex consists of many closely related bacterial species and sub-species (Figure 2.4). Among these include *M. tuberculosis sensu stricto* and *M. africanum* which are adapted to humans, together with several forms adapted to animals, for instance *M. bovis* [164]. Additionally, *M. canettii* is characterized by a more distinct smooth tuberculosis bacilli or colony morphology [165-167]. Interestingly, the genetic population structure of a group of *M.tb* strains harbours a deletion in the *M.tb* genomic region known as TBD1 (referred to as evolutionarily "modern") compared to *M.tb* strains without TBD1 (referred to as evolutionarily "ancestral" or "ancient") [168]. Currently, based on WGS analyses, the *M.tb* global phylogeny consists of seven lineages (L1 to L7) (Figure 2.4) [169]. A more recent 2020 publication identified Lineage 8 (L8); an as-yet-unknown lineage that needs to be investigated further [170].

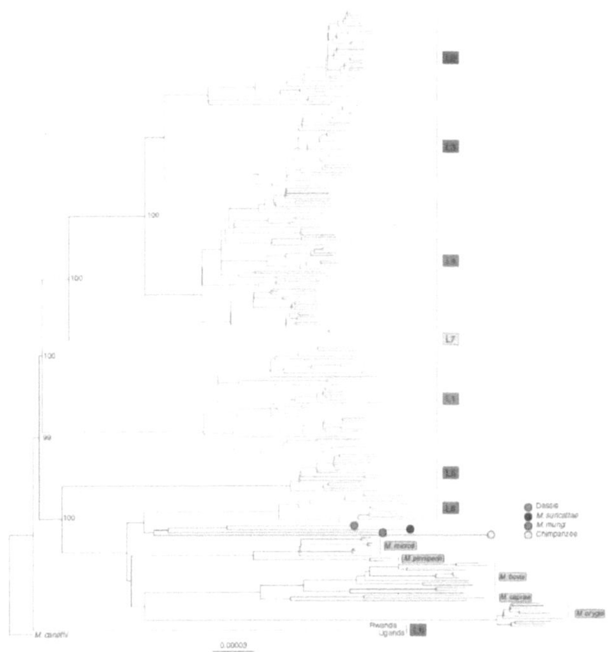


Nagabonziza *et al.* [170]

**Figure 2. 4** Maximum likelihood phylogeny of 241 *M.tb* genomes, inferred from 43 442 variable positions

**Note:** Scale bar shows the number of substitutions per polymorphic site. Human-adapted strains are indicated by coloured branches, whereas animal-adapted strains are indicated in black. The phylogeny rooted on *M. canettii* and shows the distribution of *M.tb* adapted lineages 1 to 8 (L1-L8)

Lineage 2, 3 and 4 belongs to the "modern" TBD1 deleted monophyletic group, whereas the remaining lineages belong to the "ancestral" paraphyletic group (do not comprise of a single phylogenetic group). Several studies suggest that these *M.tb* lineages are confined to certain geographical settings (some more widespread than others); thus, showing a strong phylogeographic population structure [113, 117, 171-175]. Many studies explored the most globally widespread groups, namely Lineage 2 (East Asian) and Lineage 4 (Euro-American) strain families [154, 176-179], but few studies explored the remaining strain families [156, 158].

East Africa and certain parts of Asia (Central, South and South-East Asia) comprise mainly of Lineage 1 and 3; whereas Lineage 2 (East Asian lineage) includes Beijing strains and predominates in East Asia, but has also been reported in Central Asia, Russia and South Africa [180]. Lineage 4 (Euro-American lineage) mostly originates in Asia, Europe, America and Africa; whereas lineage 5 to 7 originates in specific regions within Africa [169]. For instance, lineage 5 and 6 is often referred to as *M. africanum* West Africa 1 and 2, respectively, originating in West Africa or among recent immigrants from these areas [169]. More recently, lineage 7 is restricted to Ethiopia and Ethiopian immigrants only [181], whereas Lineage 8 seems to be restricted to the African Great Lakes region in the eastern part of the African continent [170].

Mycobacteria also exists in different animal (wild or domestic) species. The first of these lineages includes the following animal associated strains: *M. bovis* (including the BCG vaccine strains), *M. caprae* (goats, sheep), *M. microti* (voles), *M. origys* (antelopes) and *M. pinnipedii* (seal and sea lions). The second lineage of strains that is associated with animals includes the chimpanzee bacillus, the dassie bacillis (hyrax), *M. mungi* (banded mongooses) and *M. suricatae* (meerkats); sharing a common ancestor with lineage 6 strains [182-185]. Lastly, ancient *M.tb* peruvian human strains, were found in 1000 year old human remains from Peru. These strains were very much different to any of the human adapted *M.tb*, yet closely linked to *M. pinnipedii*; suggesting transmission of marine mammals across the ocean to various settings (Figure 2.4) [186]. Interestingly, among these animal strains, a deletion of the genomic region of difference 1 (RD1) first described in BCG [187], originated in the genomes of *M. microti, M. mungi* and the dassie bacillus [115, 183, 188].

In summary, WGS has a greater advantage over other genotyping methods, with the ability to define transmission clusters during outbreaks (including strain diversity), by combining genomic and epidemiological data in order to detect and interpret novel resistance conferring mutations, and/or mechanisms for all TB drugs [127, 128]. Thus, WGS could predict DR-TB phenotypes and may help guide clinicians with TB treatment for patients [129].

# CHAPTER THREE

# 3. Methodology

## 3.1 Study setting and design

Khayelitsha is a peri-urban township situated 40 kilometres from the City of Cape Town. Surrounding areas in Khayelitsha include Macassar, Eerste river, Blue downs and Mitchells Plain (Figure 3.1).

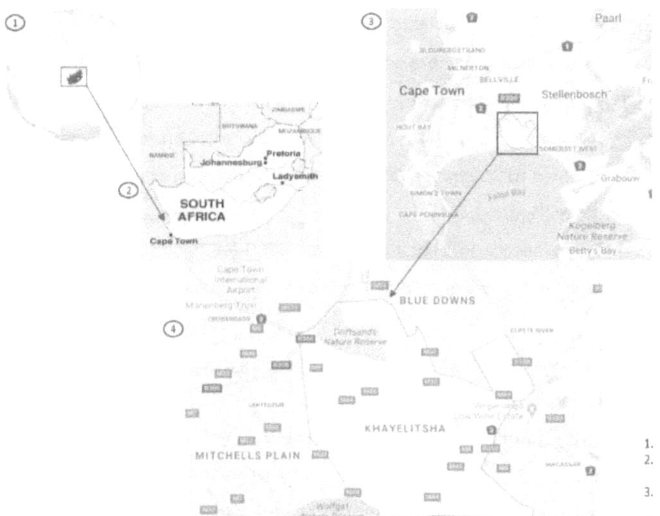


1. Global view of South Africa
2. Cape Town in the Western Cape Province, South Africa
3. Khayelitsha located on the Cape Flats, Cape Town
4. Khayelitsha and surrounding areas

Adapted from: google maps

**Figure 3. 1** Maps illustrating the location of this study setting, Khayelitsha, located on the Cape Flats in Cape Town, the Western Cape Province, South Africa

In 2011, Khayelitsha had an estimated population of 400 000 individuals, half of whom live in informal housing settlements, facing a high rate of poverty and unemployment [189]. There are eight primary care clinics and three large community health centres in the Khayelitsha subdistrict that provide TB, drug-resistant TB (DR-TB), and HIV diagnosis and treatment. In 2011, the TB case notification rate was at least 1500 per 100 000 people per year in Khayelitsha [190-192]. Recent data from 2019; the Western Cape Provincial Health Department; reported an estimated 74 252 adults who were HIV positive (>15 years), of whom 44 583 were on antiretroviral treatment (ART) for HIV, in Khayelitsha [193]. According to a survey done in Khayelitsha during 2008, RR-TB was found among 4.5% new and

11.2% previously TB treated cases [43]. In late 2007, a programme was implemented in Khayelitsha by Médecins sans Frontières (MSF) in partnership with the City of Cape Town and the Western Cape Province Government to provide decentralized community-based DR-TB treatment [192]. Decentralisation was based on patient-centred care and treatment with principles such as individual rifampicin-resistant TB (RR-TB) counselling, routine home visits, family education, patient support groups, and contact tracing and screening. Hospitalisation occurred only if patients were clinically unstable and/or unable to attend their clinic for daily treatment. The programme was associated with increases in DR-TB case detection and the proportion of diagnosed patients starting treatment, along with a reduction in delays to treatment initiation. However, proportional treatment success remained poor despite the community-based DR-TB programme [194].

Since the GeneXpert MTB/RIF (Xpert) test was implemented in late 2011, there has been no significant increase in DR-TB case detection. Before 2011, drug susceptibility testing (DST) was only available for individuals with presumptive TB who had a history of previous TB treatment or were at high-risk for DR-TB. After 2012, the Xpert test was given to all individuals with presumptive TB. Due to poor treatment outcomes, particularly among multi-drug resistant TB (MDR-TB) patients, an additional programme was implemented in Khayelitsha from 2012 to provide new and repurposed drugs into strengthened regimens. These drugs comprise of linezolid (repurposed drug), bedaquiline and delamanid (newer TB drugs). Studies have shown improved treatment outcomes using these drugs [195, 196].

## 3.2 Ethical considerations

This study is embedded within a broader study of a systems approach to evaluate prospects for the control of DR-TB in Khayelitsha, South Africa. The broader study [HREC/REF: 416/2014], as well as this doctoral research study [HREC/REF: 845/2016], has been previously submitted and approved at the Research Ethics Committee at the University of Cape Town (UCT). This includes approval to link TB isolate genotype data to clinical data, to conduct whole genome sequencing (WGS), and to contribute WGS and anonymised meta-data to data-sharing platforms.

Laboratory specimen numbers were used to link patients between databases. Once linkage was completed and data was validated, all patient identifying data were removed, and study identification numbers were used to identify individuals. Confidentiality of data was always considered during the study. All data repositories were password protected, with access only by listed study investigators. If previously unidentified drug resistance was detected during this study and the patient remained in care, the information was forwarded to the treating clinician.

## 3.3 Data sources

### 3.3.1 Biobank of RR-TB isolates

All RR-TB isolates derived from specimens routinely submitted to the National Health Laboratory Service (NHLS) from the Western Cape Province, South Africa, are stored in a biobank at the Division of Molecular Biology and Human Genetics, Faculty of Medicine and Health Sciences at Stellenbosch University (SU). The broader Khayelitsha study aims to utilise clinical data and stored *M.tb* isolates from the biobank across the period 2008-2017 (Figure 3.2). For the purpose of this book, clinical data and stored *M.tb* isolates from the biobank are utilized from a more recent subset from the broader study, i.e. across 2013-2015 inclusive (Chapter 6 to 9). Only data from Chapter 5 includes the overall prevalence among RR-TB patients diagnosed in Khayelitsha (from the broader study) across the period 2008-2017 inclusive.

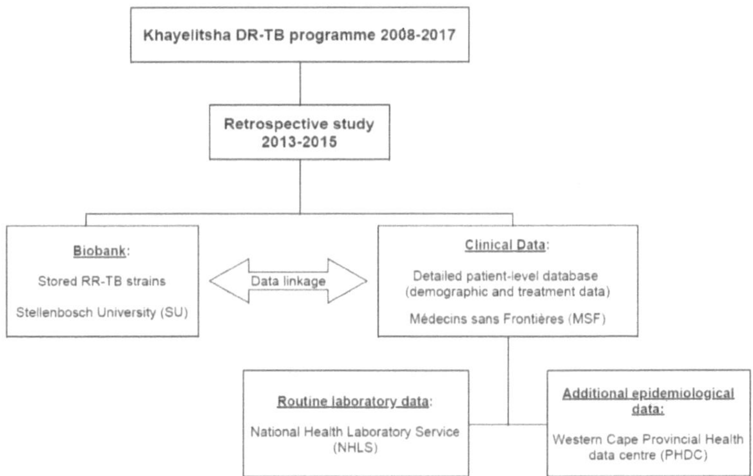


**Figure 3. 2** Diagrammatic representation of data linkage in this study

### 3.3.2 Clinical data

The MSF Khayelitsha programme supports operational research and maintains high quality routine clinical data collection from 2008. Data on an individual patient level such as demographic, clinical and treatment information are recorded. There are approximately 200 patients diagnosed with RR-TB per year in Khayelitsha. Data from TB related laboratory records from the NHLS are also recorded on a routine basis. As part of the broader study, the clinical database has been linked to the biobank of stored rifampicin mono-resistant TB (RMR-TB) and MDR-TB strains at SU.

### 3.3.3 Additional epidemiological data

Data on previous first-line TB treatment for RR-TB patients diagnosed from 2013-2015 were obtained from the Western Cape Provincial Health Data Centre (PHDC). The PHDC collates data from a range of different data sources, including the electronic tuberculosis register (ETR), the DR-TB register (EDRweb), routine HIV and ART registers, laboratory and pharmaceutical supply data [197].

We retrospectively assessed whether individuals were previously treated for TB and whether they were HIV positive during that previous first-line TB treatment by using PHDC data on TB and HIV episodes. We also determined whether these individuals were receiving ART during previous TB treatment. Relative proportions of RMR- to MDR-TB were then assessed among the various categories.

## 3.4 Sample selection

Based on routine data from Khayelitsha, RMR-TB isolates accounted for approximately 18% of all RR-TB cases from 2005-2011 [192]. The percentages of RMR- and MDR-TB from 2008-2017, and during the study period, remained relatively stable at approximately 20% and 80%, respectively. Chapter 5 (Epidemiology of RMR-TB in Khayelitsha) contains details of RR-TB patients routinely diagnosed in Khayelitsha.

## 3.5 Overview of workflow

All laboratory techniques involving the handling of live *M.tb* cultures were done in the Biosafety Level 3 (BSL3) laboratory at the Division of Molecular Biology and Human Genetics, 4$^{th}$ floor, Fisan building, Faculty of Medicine and Health Sciences, SU. Strict BSL3 safety procedures were taken into consideration to prevent contamination of bacterial cultures or human exposure to mycobacterial cultures. Refer to figure 3.3 for a diagrammatic representation of the general workflow in this study.

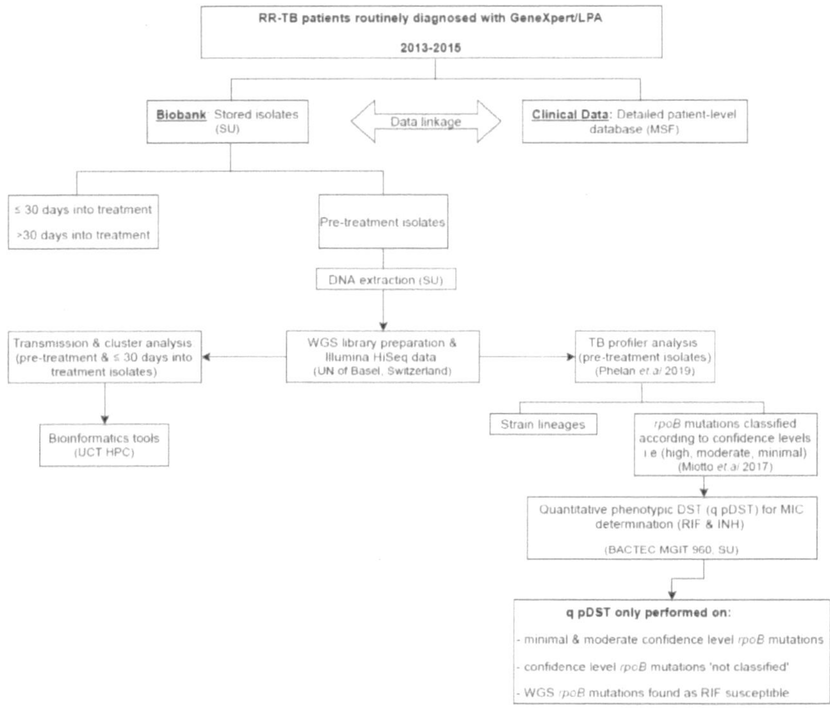


**Figure 3. 3** General overview of the workflow for the cohort of RR-TB during 2013-15

In this study, the phrase "RR-TB patients routinely diagnosed" refers to the initial, routine National Health Laboratory Service (NHLS) results. *M.tb* clinical isolates with routine RR-TB results with either the GenoType MTBDR*plus* line probe assay (LPA) and/or the Xpert (Cepheid, Sunnyvale, USA) were collected, stored and retrospectively retrieved from the biobank at SU. Retrieved isolates were either pre-treatment; or isolates from patients taken ≤30 days or >30 days into treatment. WGS was performed to determine mutations in the *rpoB* gene that conferred rifampicin resistance (RIF R), and to detect potential transmission clusters. A detailed description of all these steps will follow.

Briefly, stored frozen cultures were sub-cultured into mycobacterial growth indicator tubes (MGITs) for the process of DNA extraction (refer to section 3.6 and 3.7). DNA was extracted at SU and sent to the University of Basel in Switzerland for library preparation and WGS of isolates on the Illumina HiSeq. After gathering WGS data, TB profiler was used to identify resistance-conferring mutations in the *rpoB* gene, and strain lineages were identified [141]. Mutations in the *rpoB* region were further classified as high, moderate and minimal confidence in conferring RIF R based on the criteria described by

Miotto *et al.* [147]. The *Escherichia coli (E. coli)* gene nomenclature for naming *rpoB* mutations was used throughout this study [20, 23]. Quantitative phenotypic drug susceptibility testing (q pDST) was performed for isolates with minimal, moderate and *rpoB* confidence level mutations that were not classified by Miotto *et al.* [147]. Additionally, q pDST was performed on WGS derived isolates found to be rifampicin susceptible TB (RS-TB) [no RIF R conferring *rpoB* mutations detected] but were isolated from patients routinely diagnosed with RR-TB. For transmission cluster analysis, WGS data was analysed with various bioinformatics tools. Computations were performed using facilities provided by UCT's Information and Communication Technology Services (ICTS) High Performance Computing (HPC) team (Refer to section 3.11). One isolate per patient was included, either a pre-treatment isolate, or if not available, an isolate from a specimen taken ≤30 days into treatment. We excluded stored isolates of patients from routine sputum samples that were taken >30 days into treatment. The reason for this was that we wanted to capture recent transmission within newly diagnosed RR-TB cases (as defined by the WHO 2016) [3].

## 3.6 Storage and Identification of isolates

*M.tb* isolates were stored in Nunc cryovials containing polypropylene glass beads (with peptone) for subculture from the selected sample isolated. Each cryovial was labelled according to the allocated study numbers. After inoculation, each cryovial was stored at -80°C until further testing. This method was conducted aseptically and according to the instructions by the manufacturer.

For sub-culturing of frozen cultures, MGIT tubes containing 7 ml of modified Middlebrook 7H9 broth base; were labelled with specimen numbers followed by the addition of 0.8 ml of reconstituted PANTA (Polymyxin B, Amphotericin B, Nalidixic Acid, Trimethoprim, Azlocillin) /enrichment growth supplement. Two single glass beads coated with *M.tb* (selected isolates) from frozen Nunc cryovials were added to the corresponding MGIT tube. Inoculated MGIT tubes were scanned and placed into the BACTEC MGIT 960 instrument. MGIT tubes were incubated at 37°C until the instrument flagged the tubes positive. After these MGIT tubes flagged positive, 0.25 ml of sub-cultured MGIT (containing PANTA with glass beads) was inoculated into a fresh MGIT tube; containing 0.8 ml of OADC (Oleic acid, albumin, dextrose and catalase) growth supplement; and further incubated at 37°C until the instrument flagged the tubes positive. This suspension of MGIT tubes was either used for DNA extraction or q pDST (re-cultured at different time points).

## 3.7 DNA extraction

All selected *M.tb* isolates were cultured, and total genomic DNA was extracted in preparation for WGS. The DNA extraction procedure was carried out according to the protocol by Warren *et al.* [198] and was conducted at the Division of Molecular Biology and Human Genetics, Faculty of Medicine and Health Science at SU. This process took approximately three days (excluding tissue culture growth) including stages such as denaturation of proteins and RNA, as well as precipitation of DNA.

Mycobacterial cultivation occurred in the MGIT tube containing Middlebrook OADC supplement media under BSL3 conditions. After the tissue culture was grown sufficiently, 500 µl (from the MGIT tube) was transferred to a 7H11 plate and incubated at 37°C for approximately 21 days. Once sufficient growth was observed on the plate, heat inactivation of *M.tb* cultures occurred by incubating plates in a pre-heated fan oven at 80°C for ~1.5 to 2 hours. Meanwhile, 6 ml extraction buffer (5% sodium glutamate, 50 mM Tris-HCl [pH 7.4] and 25 mM EDTA) was added to its corresponding labelled polypropylene Falcon tube (50 ml) containing 20 glass beads (diameter, 5 mm). Thereafter, bacteria from the media were carefully scraped off using a sterile disposable 10µl plastic loop to transfer into the corresponding labelled 50 ml Falcon tube which were vigorously vortexed for 2 minutes. Lysozyme (500 µl) [100 mg/ml; Roche, Germany] and RNase A (2.5 µl) [10 mg/ml; Roche, Germany] were added to each bacterial suspension, with an incubation period of 2 hours at 37°C after gentle mixing. Afterwards, 600 µl of 10x proteinase K buffer (5% sodium dodecyl sulfate, 100 mM Tris-HCl [pH 7.8], 50 mM EDTA) and 300 µl of proteinase K enzyme (10 mg/ml; Roche, Germany) were added for the denaturation of proteins. The suspension was gently mixed and incubated at 45°C for 16 hours.

An equal volume of phenol-chloroform-isoamyl alcohol (25/24/1) was added (in a standard fume cabinet) and intermittently mixed (every 30 minutes) over a period of 2 hours at room temperature. For complete phase separation, centrifugation at 3000 rpm for 20 minutes at room temperature was performed. The initial aqueous phase was carefully aspirated; without collecting interface; and transferred into a clean 50 ml falcon tube containing 5 ml of chloroform/isoamyl alcohol (24:1). Thereafter, tubes were once more subjected to centrifugation at 3000 rpm for 20 minutes at room temperature. The resultant aqueous phase was carefully aspirated, without collecting interface, and transferred into a clean 50 ml falcon tube containing 600 µl 3 M sodium acetate (pH 5.2). Next, the DNA was precipitated by adding 7 ml ice cold isopropanol with immediate collection on a thin glass rod. The glass rod containing the DNA was washed in a 1.5 ml tube containing 70% ethanol (1 ml) with a 10 minute incubation period. Thereafter, the glass rod with precipitated DNA was transferred to a new labelled 1.5 ml tube and incubated at room temperature until the DNA was dry (minimum 2-3 hours). Lastly, the DNA was rehydrated by adding 300 µl-600 µl TE (pH 8), releasing the DNA from the glass rod by gently mixing. The DNA was left to re-dissolve by overnight incubation at 4°C or for 2 hours at 65°C. The DNA was stored at -20°C until further use.

### 3.7.1 DNA quality

DNA quality checks were conducted at the Division of Molecular Biology and Human Genetics, Faculty of Medicine and Health Science at SU. Firstly, DNA concentrations were measured with the Nanodrop ND-1000 Spectrophotometer instrument according to the manufacturer's instructions (Nanodrop Technologies, Inc., Wilmington, DE, USA). Briefly, a spectrophotometer is an instrument measuring the number of molecules that absorb a specific wavelength of energy. The nanodrop can analyse 1 to 2 µl samples of either DNA, RNA, proteins, dyes or microbial cell culture. In this instance, nucleic acid of 2 µl was used. Blank measurements were made in between each DNA measurement with the addition of 2 µl nuclease free water (Promega, Madison, USA) to prevent inaccurate sample readings. An optical density (OD) of 1 at 260 nm was equivalent to 50 µg/µl of double-stranded DNA. The purity of DNA was assessed by observing the partnership of values between $OD_{260}/OD_{280}$. These partner values were between 1.8 and 2.0.

Secondly, gel electrophoresis was performed to confirm DNA purity and size on agarose gels. A 1% agarose gel was prepared with 3 g of Seakem LE agarose gel powder (Whitehead Scientific) and 300 ml 1xTBE buffer. For the gels, ethidium bromide was used (10mg/ml stock diluted 2.5 µl/100 ml TBE). After gel solidification, the gel was placed into a gel tank with 1xTBE buffer. The buffer provides continuous flow of the electric current during electrophoresis and prevents melting of the gel. For each sample, 1 µl DNA were mixed with 1 µl blue/orange 6x loading buffer (Promega, Madison, USA) and together loaded with a pipette into individual wells of the gel. After connecting the negative and positive electrodes to the PowerPac Basic supply box (Bio-Rad, France), the gel was run at 100 volts for approximately 2 hours. After gel electrophoresis, the gel was carefully placed in a UV machine to visualize the DNA bands with the GelDoc computer system (Bio-Rad, France). All DNA bands were viewed to ensure DNA purity of each sample before sending the DNA to Switzerland for WGS.

## 3.8 Whole genome sequencing

Following DNA quality checks, genomic DNA of each sample were sent to Switzerland for WGS using the Illumina HiSeq 2000 instrument with 100 or 115 cycles and an expected coverage of 100x. This instrument is available at the joint core Genomics Facility of the University of Basel and ETH Zurich at the D-BSSE in Basel and includes robotics for fast and cost-effective sample preparation. Library preparation (300 base pair (bp) paired-end library) for each purified DNA sample was performed in Switzerland, followed by sequencing.

After the completion of sequencing, the raw fastq WGS data files of the sequenced DNA were provided by the University of Basel, Switzerland Tropical and Public Health Institute. The data was shared in South Africa via a secure network via UCT filesender (http://filesend.uct.ac.za) for external collaborators to upload large raw data files for download. These data files were stored on an external hard-drive and processed on UCT's HPC cluster (http://hpc.uct.ac.za/).

### 3.8.1 Whole genome sequencing analysis

TB profiler, developed at the London School of Hygiene and Tropical Medicine, is an online tool established in 2015, to report drug resistance and strain lineages directly from raw sequence data [142]. TB profiler also allows profiling through a Unix, command line interface. Recently, a new updated version of TB profiler was released by Phelan *et al.* [141] to allow profiling with additional functionality such as batch processing of samples, and the ability to process minION data. Additionally, report outputs are written in *json, txt* and *pdf* formats, with the option of collating data into multi-sample reports. In this study, the updated version was used for WGS analysis and data was processed locally through a command line environment to obtain outputs [141].

TB profiler uses a perl script to apply the *Snap* software and *samtool/vcf* based bioinformatic pipeline (Figure 3.4). Briefly, reads are trimmed using trimmomatic, followed by the alignment of reads to the reference genome using burrows-wheeler transform algorithm (BWA) or minimap2 for nanopore. Thereafter, variants are called using genome analysis toolkit (GATK). Refer to section 3.11 on transmission cluster analysis for more details on these bioinformatic tools.

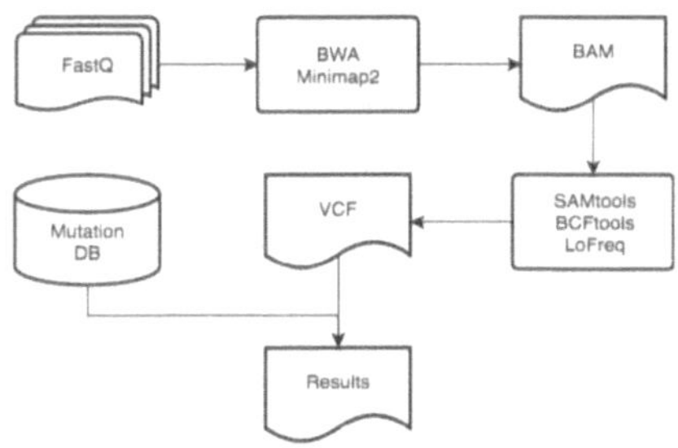


Phelan *et al.* [141]

**Figure 3. 4** Bioinformatics pipeline used for TB profiler

The pipeline reads small variants and big deletions associated with drug resistance and reports strain lineages. Coll *et al.* [142] compiled a library of 1,325 drug resistance markers and developed the TB profiler online tool in Perl/PHP. To characterise mutations from WGS files (*fastq* format), raw sequences were mapped to a modified version of the H37Rv reference genome (Genbank accession number: NC_000962.3) by using the *Snap* algorithm [199]. Single nucleotide polymorphism (SNPs) and indels were called using *samtool/vcf* tools of high quality (Q30, 1 error per 1,000 bp) [200, 201]. The modified reference genome contains genes and regional sequences of drug resistance mutations and selected lineage specific mutations [200]. The library included the following anti-TB drugs: rifampicin (RIF), isoniazid (INH), ethambutol, ethionamide, pyrazinamide, streptomycin and second line drugs amikacin, capreomycin, kanamycin, moxifloxin, ofloxacin. Additionally, para-aminosalicylic acid, linezolid, clofazimine and bedaquiline were added to the library. Known and novel polymorphisms were determined by comparing high quality SNPs and indels identified from the alignments to the curated list. The new version of TB profiler mutation library was updated to include 178 new mutations, including additional drugs, cycloserine and delamanid, that were not present in the previous version of the library [141].

## 3.9 Quantitative phenotypic drug susceptibility testing: MGIT 960

### 3.9.1 Strain selection and drug concentrations

Following WGS, a subset of RMR- and MDR-TB strains with minimal, moderate or 'non classified' confidence level *rpoB* mutations as per WGS results were selected. Following identification of isolates, q pDST was performed for RIF and INH drugs using the MGIT 960 system as recommended by the manufacturer (Becton, Dickinson, Sparks, MD). Critical drug concentrations were applied at 1.0 µg/ml for RIF. INH resistance was tested with low (0.1 µg/ml) and high (1 µg/ml) level minimal inhibitory concentrations (MICs). RIF MICs were determined at doubling drug concentrations ranging from 0.03 to 1.0 µg/ml, including 2.0, 6.0, 10 and 20 µg/ml (Table 3.1) [28, 202]. Also, WGS-derived results that showed no *rpoB* mutations (RS-TB) but were isolated from patients routinely diagnosed with RR-TB were further tested with q pDST (Table 3.1). Quality control (QC) was performed on each batch of reagents and drugs used. *M.tb* H37Rv (American Type Culture Collection [ATCC], number 27294) was used as a QC strain which is susceptible to all TB drugs.

**Table 3. 1** Concentrations of drugs used for MIC determination

| Drugs | Minimum inhibitory concentrations used for testing in the MGIT 960 (µg/ml) | WGS *rpoB* mutations classified by confidence levels |
|---|---|---|
| Rifampicin (RIF) | 0.03, 0.06, 0.125, 0.25, 0.5, 1.0 | Minimal |
| Rifampicin (RIF) | 1.0, 2.0, 6.0, 10, 20 | Moderate |
| Rifampicin (RIF) | 0.5, 1.0, 2.0, 6.0, 10, 20 | Not classified |
| Rifampicin (RIF) | 0.5; 1.0 | no *rpoB* mutations (RS-TB by WGS) |
| Isoniazid (INH) | 0.1, 1.0 | Minimal, moderate, 'not classified' and no *rpoB* mutations (RS-TB by WGS) |

**Note:** RR-TB isolates were classified by confidence levels (Miotto *et al.* [147]) followed by MIC testing at varying concentrations for each confidence level classification

### 3.9.2 Preparation of drug concentrations

Before setting up MGIT tubes for q pDST or MIC determination, drug stock solutions at specific concentrations are required. A final stock solution of 840 µg/ml was calculated for both drugs. For RIF, 8.4 mg of drug was dissolved in 4 ml dimethyl sulfoxide (DMSO) and 6 ml sterile distilled water, and mixed well until dissolved. For INH, 14.3 mg was dissolved in 17 ml sterile distilled water, and mixed well until dissolved. The final stock solutions for both drugs were sterilised by filtration through a syringe filter; specifically, Milex-LG 0.20 µm hydrophilic PTFE filters (Millipor Corporation); in the BSL3 laboratory. Small aliquots of final stock solutions were dispensed into labelled sterile screw-cap tubes and stored at -80°C until further required. Working solutions of 84 µg/ml were used to dilute MICs below 1 µg/ml with sterile distilled water.

### 3.9.3 Sub-culturing and inoculum preparation

All laboratory procedures were aseptically performed in the BSL3 laboratory. Following section 3.6 (Storage and identification of isolates), each isolate was sub-cultured into a MGIT tube, labelled with the specimen number. Sub-culturing included the addition of 0.8 ml MGIT growth supplement (OADC) followed by 0.25 ml of inoculum into the corresponding MGIT tube. However, sub-culturing was repeated for slow growing isolates (growth >6 days) by increasing the inoculum to 0.35 ml - 0.4 ml. Isolates that failed to grow with no bacterial growth detected after 14 days of inoculation were reported as no growth or non-viable.

The test inoculum was prepared on a positive MGIT tube after it was first identified as positive on the MGIT instrument (day 0). At day 1 or day 2, the MGIT culture was directly used for preparing the inoculum for susceptibility testing. When a MGIT tube was at day 3, 4, or 5, a 1:5 dilution (1 ml of the

MGIT culture diluted in 4 ml sterile saline) was used for preparing the inoculum for susceptibility testing.

### 3.9.4 Preparation of inoculum for q pDST

All MGIT tubes were labelled with the corresponding specimen (accession) number and drugs for testing. For each isolate, MGIT tubes included one drug-free 1:100 growth control (GC), two INH drug concentrations and the different RIF drug concentrations in correlation to the *rpoB* confidence level mutations (Table 3.1).

Every isolate was tested once, unless slow growth was observed, then the isolate was re-cultured and once more subjected to MIC testing. Specimen registration was performed on the BD EpiCenter System according to the manufacturers instructions [100]. Epi-Center labels were printed accordingly with accession numbers and attached to the corresponding isolate number on each MGIT tube.

For MIC inoculation of the MGIT tubes, 0.8 ml of MGIT growth supplement (OADC) was aseptically added; followed by 100 µl of prepared RIF and INH drugs (section 3.9.2) into the corresponding labelled MGIT tubes according to its individual MIC concentration.

Thereafter, the drug-free GC was prepared by inoculating 0.1 ml of the positive MGIT culture directly into a 10 ml sterile saline tube (1:100 dilution inoculum). The GC inoculum was thoroughly vortexed, before inoculating 0.5 ml into the corresponding GC MGIT tube. Aseptically, 0.5 ml of the positive MGIT culture was inoculated into all the MGIT tubes labelled with MICs for RIF and INH. Thereafter, all MGIT tubes were loaded into the MGIT 960 instrument with the control first, followed by drug concentration tubes in ascending order. All tubes were incubated at 37°C and results were monitored weekly on the Epi-Center [100].

### 3.9.5 Interpretation of MGIT results

For the interpretation of the MGIT results, the user manual was referred to for TB eXiST, Epi-Center [100]. In the growth control tube, a growth of >400 growth units (GUs) was reached before the machine evaluated the drug containing MGIT tubes. The MGIT 960 system monitored these growth patterns and the results were interpreted as susceptible, intermediate or resistant. An isolate was resistant when the GU reached ≥400 in the drug-free control tube, while the GU of the drug-containing tube reached ≥100. However, when the GU in the drug-containing tube was <100 after 7 days when the GC reached ≥400 GU, the isolate was defined as susceptible. If the GU of the drug-containing tube was ≥100 during a 7-day incubation period, after the GU of the drug-free control tube reached >400, the isolate was defined as intermediate [100]. After all the results were obtained, comparisons were made between MICs by q pDST, WGS resistance conferring *rpoB* mutations and the corresponding confidence levels [147].

## 3.10 Statistical analysis

All data were analysed using the IBM Statistical Package for Social Sciences (SPSS); version 25. A chi-square test was used to analyse differences in MDR-TB and RMR-TB association between test variables using SPSS. A p-value less than 0.05 was considered statistically significant. This included univariate analysis to estimate the Odds Ratio (OR) and 95% Confidence intervals (CI). Variables were entered into multivariate models based on univariate significance or presumed importance based on literature. Chi-squared analyses were used to assess trends over time.

## 3.11 Transmission cluster analysis

Strain lineages and mutations were identified using TB profiler through command line [141]. The WGS pipeline for the analysis of transmission events were established in collaboration between UCT (South Africa) and the University of Basel (Switzerland). The pipeline shows how SNPs are produced from raw Illumina sequence data. A combination of software packages was used, as well as in-house developed scripts to compile a pipeline for transmission cluster analysis (Figure 3.5).

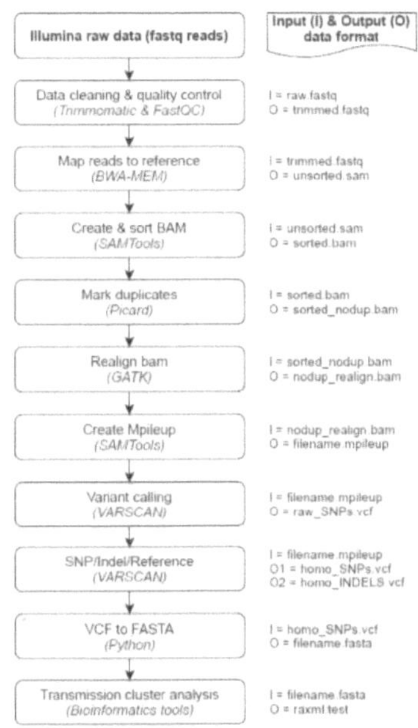


**Figure 3. 5** The summarised workflow of bioinformatics tools used for whole genome sequencing data for phylogeny analysis

### 3.11.1 Fastq file format

A fastq sequence file (raw sequencing data) is a text-based format for storing biological sequences such as a nucleotide sequence and its corresponding quality score information as provided by the sequencing instrument [203]. Fastq files are either run as single-reads containing one Read 1 (R1) or paired-end reads containing one R1 and one Read 2 (R2) fastq files.

### 3.11.2 Data cleaning and quality control

Trimmomatic version 0.39 (phred +33) was used to remove possible contaminating Illumina adapter sequences (trimming of reads) and bad quality bases. Adapter contamination could result in next generation sequencing (NGS) alignment errors and an increased number of unaligned reads, since adapter sequences are synthetic and does not appear in the genomic sequence. This step improved the overall average quality of the results by improving mapping to the *M.tb* ancestor reference genome. It also reduced the number of false positive SNP calls [204].

FastQC version 0.11.8 was used to check the overall quality of sequence reads. Isolates with a quality of reads (coverage) above 20 were included [205].

### 3.11.3 Alignment and mapping

BWA; version 0.7.17, was used to map the single or paired trimmed sequencing reads (trimmed.fastq) to the *M.tb* ancestor reference genome by using *bwa-mem*. BWA produces a mapping file in a sequence alignment map (SAM) format that contains all the information for downstream analyses. However, the size of SAM files makes it difficult to work with. Thus, another format called binary alignment map (BAM); a binary version of a SAM file; was used instead [206].

### 3.11.4 SAMTools, Picard and GATK

SAMTools version 1.9 was used to produce BAM, which is the binary format of SAM files. Thereafter, the BAM files were sorted by position ready for variant calling. Duplicates can arise during library construction using PCR amplification. The Picard command "MarkDuplicates" was used to identify duplicate reads in the BAM file, which were flagged in the output BAM file [207]. Thereafter, GATK; version 3.5, was used for re-alignment of the bam file. Once more, SAMTools was used to create a "mpileup" file before identifying SNPs.

### 3.11.5 VarScan and Python

VarScan makes consensus calls (SNP/Indel/Reference) from the "mpileup" file, based on user-defined parameters [208]. These parameters included variants with at least 5 reads in both strains; and a minimum read depth of 7. A quality score/coverage of 20 was selected where 10% of reads supported the variant allele.

The variant call format (VCF) file produced by SAMTools contains information about the genomic position, the reference base, the number of reads covering the site, read bases and base qualities [209]. A python script was used to convert the VCF to fasta files; used as input for further transmission cluster analysis (section 3.11.6). SNPs with ≥90% frequency were included to detect recent transmission [120, 210]. Lastly, SNPs annotated in regions that were difficult to map, for instance, repetitive elements (PPE/PE-PGRS, Maturase, Phage) were removed from analysis [211]; also those detected in a window of 10 variants near indels [120].

### 3.11.6 Transmission cluster analysis

Randomised Axelerated Maximum Likelihood (RAxML); version 8, was used for phylogenetic construction [212]. Phylogenetic trees were visualized using FigTree; version 1.4.3. The program has a graphical interface to modify components of the tree; such as rooting positions, node labels, tip labels and scale axes [213].

Clusterpicker; version 1.2.5, was used to identify genomic clusters found among RR-TB strains (RMR- and MDR-TB), to infer recent transmission by generating a phylogenetic tree. Outputs were strain lineages, as well as RMR- and MDR-TB included within the phylogenetic tree [214]. Even though many SNP cut-offs for linking isolates have previously been proposed [63], the most frequently used is a SNP threshold of 12 for inferring possible transmission between TB cases [156, 162]. For this reason, a SNP threshold of 12 was used in this study, according to Walker *et al.* [156]. In other words, genomic clusters were defined with no more than 12 SNPs separating a patient isolate from at least one other patient in a cluster.

Lastly, an R script was used for generating a distance matrix for SNP pairwise comparison. The output gave the exact SNP differences between all genomes within clustered and non-clustered groups. Where applicable, a minimum spanning tree was manually drawn to visualise possible transmission between patients.

# CHAPTER FOUR

# 4. Temporal trends, transmission and risk factors associated with rifampicin mono-resistant tuberculosis: a systematic review

## 4.1 Introduction

Rifampicin mono-resistant tuberculosis (RMR-TB) comprises 22% and 38% of all rifampicin-resistant TB (RR-TB) globally and in South Africa, respectively [2]. Previously, rifampicin resistance (RIF R) was said to be a proxy for multidrug-resistant TB (MDR-TB; defined as rifampicin and isoniazid resistance) because of prior reports of high correlations between RIF R and MDR-TB [215]. In the past, observations were made that isoniazid mono-resistant TB (HMR-TB) was more common than RMR-TB [12, 216], leading to the assumption that MDR-TB occurs through the initial acquisition of isoniazid (INH) resistance first, followed by RIF R.

Previously, estimates of the drug-resistant TB (DR-TB) burden from World Health Organization (WHO) global TB reports focused mainly on MDR-TB. However, the WHO global TB report of 2016 [217] reported on all RR-TB, including MDR-TB (referring to MDR/RR-TB in the report). According to the WHO global TB report of 2019, it was reported that an estimated 484 000 incident cases of MDR/RR-TB occurred globally in 2018, and that approximately 22% (136 000) of these were RMR-TB [2].

Previous analyses using data from 14 supranational TB reference laboratories across 2000 to 2004, reported wide variation in the prevalence of RMR-TB among all RR-TB isolates, ranging from 0.5% in the Middle East to 11.6% in Korea [218]. Furthermore, global data from 81 countries on anti-TB drug resistance surveillance from 1994 to 2007, showed that as the MDR-TB prevalence among all TB increased, the percentage of RMR-TB isolates among RR-TB tended to decrease (43.3% of RR-TB isolates were INH susceptible in low MDR-TB prevalence TB cohorts compared to 14% RMR-TB in high MDR-TB burden settings) [219].

Despite the above, detailed reports describing RMR-TB prevalence are limited on a global basis, especially in African countries. Data suggest that RMR-TB among all TB cases is increasing over time in the nine provinces of South Africa [4]. There are a range of factors that may contribute to the high burden of RMR-TB worldwide and several earlier studies suggest that HIV is associated with the emergence of RIF R during TB treatment. Hence, we conducted a systematic review to describe the available data on temporal trends, transmission and risk factors associated with RMR-TB.

## 4.2 Methods

### 4.2.1 Search strategy

This systematic review used the Preferred Reporting Items for Systematic reviews and Meta-Analyses; the (PRISMA) statement [220]. A search strategy with specific keywords used in combination was conducted using four electronic databases (Table 4.1). Advanced search terms were used for keywords (Table 4.1). Databases searched were PubMed, EBSCOHost-Africa, Scopus and Web of Science. The databases included within EBSCOHost-Africa were Academic Search Premier, Africa-Wide information, CINAHL, Health Source: Nursing/Academic Edition and PsycINFO. All citations were imported into the referencing software manager EndnoteX7 (Clarivate Analytics, Philadelphia, PA, USA). The literature search was conducted from 1st January 1990 until 1st April 2019.

**Table 4. 1** Key word search strategy

| Databases | Keywords |
|---|---|
| Pubmed,<br>EBSCOHost,<br>Scopus,<br>Web of Science | rifampicin mono resistant tuberculosis OR rifampin mono resistant tuberculosis OR rifamycin mono resistant tuberculosis OR RMR-TB OR isoniazid susceptibility OR RMR OR RMP OR rifampicin resistant tuberculosis<br>AND<br>risk factors OR contributing factors OR predisposing factors OR trends OR developments OR transmission OR acquisition |

**Note:** RMP (rifampicin) was included in the search as it is an alternative abbreviation used in some articles to describe RMP mono resistant tuberculosis

### 4.2.2 Study Selection

Figure 4.1 (in results section 4.3.1), summarizes the study selection process. All duplicate articles were removed. Titles and abstracts of studies were screened. The full text of potentially eligible articles was reviewed, and eligibility criteria applied. Articles were included if they presented data or descriptive findings on any one of the following i) temporal trends in RMR-TB, ii) transmission of RMR-TB, or iii) risk factors specific to RMR-TB.

Available studies on children and adults were included. Data were recorded and extracted using an excel spreadsheet. Data was extracted by Zubeida Salaam-Dreyer (ZSD); where there was uncertainty in data to be extracted, data were checked by Helen Cox (HC). Extracted information were tabulated into the above mentioned categories i) to iii), and further categorised into high and low HIV prevalence countries according to data provided by the Joint nations programme on HIV/AIDS (UNAIDS) during 2018 [221].

### 4.2.3 Terminology used in this review

RMR-TB was defined as resistance to RIF and susceptibility to INH regardless of other TB drug resistance [217]. MDR-TB was defined as resistance to both RIF and INH, also regardless of other TB drug resistance.

Articles included in this systematic review described RMR-TB in various ways. Firstly, RMR-TB was either described as a percentage of all RR-TB or as a percentage of all TB cases. Secondly, for studies that did not explicitly mention RMR-TB, the percentage of RMR-TB among all TB cases was calculated, by subtracting the percentage of MDR-TB from the percentage of RR-TB.

A new TB case was defined as a patient who had never been on TB treatment, or had taken <1 month of TB drugs previously. A previously treated TB case was defined as a patient who had received ≥ 1 month of anti-TB drugs in the past [217].

## 4.3 Results

### 4.3.1 Characteristics of identified studies

The systematic search of the four electronic databases resulted in 2492 articles (Figure 4.1). After removing duplicate studies and assessment of titles and abstracts, 115 full-text articles were screened. A total of 25 studies were considered eligible for the descriptive analysis. Temporal trends, transmission and risk factors of RMR-TB were tabulated separately (Table 4.2; 4.3; 4.4).

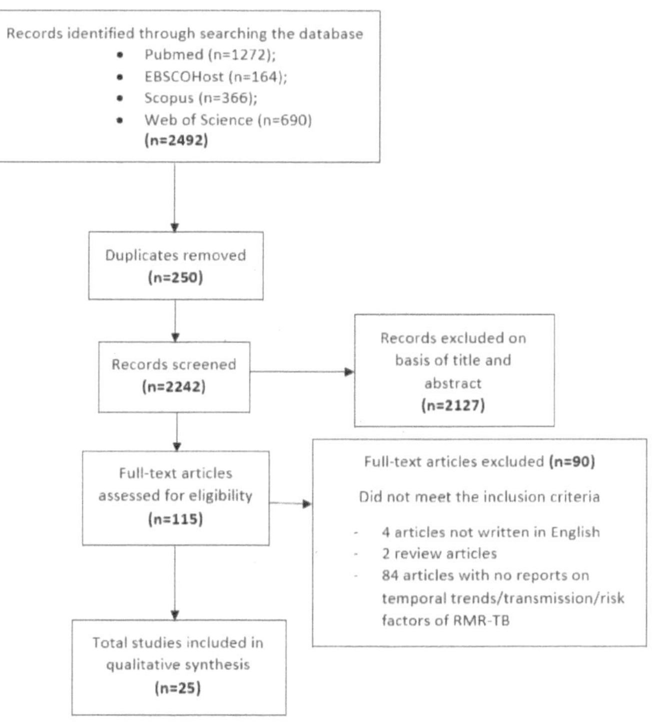


**Figure.4. 1** Flow diagram of the selection process of total studies included

**Table 4. 2** Temporal trends of RMR-TB found in 13/25 (52%) eligible studies

| Reference | Country & Region | Type of Study | Study period | Sample size | Temporal trends in RMR-TB (Summary) |
|---|---|---|---|---|---|
| ***High HIV prevalence countries*** | | | | | |
| Coovadia *et al.* [89] | Durban, KZN province, South Africa; WHO African region | Retrospective analysis of laboratory data | 2007-09 | 1466 RMR-TB (8.8%) among 16748 RR-TB | No trend; quarterly RMR-TB among RR-TB varied from 7.3% to 10% |
| Dramowski *et al.* [222] | Cape Town, Western Cape Province, South Africa; WHO African region | Prospective, single hospital-based description of childhood RMR-TB | 2003-09 | 18 children with RMR-TB | Increase; increasing number per year, ranging from 0 in 2003 to 8 in 2008/09 (16,89% 2006-08) |
| Ismail *et al.* [4] | South Africa; WHO African region | Cross-sectional, national survey, and comparison with previous survey | 2012-14 (compared to 2001-02) | RMR-TB (2.5%) among 10044 TB in 2012 | Increase; increasing from 0.4% RMR-TB among TB in 2001-02 to 3.3% in 2012-14 (statistical significance not reported) |
| Menzies *et al.* [223] | Botswana, Africa; WHO African region | Cross-sectional, national survey, and comparison with previous surveys | 2007-08 (compared to 1995-96, 1999 & 2002) | 18 RMR-TB (1.7%) among 1061 TB (2007-08) | No trend; 1.1% RMR-TB among TB in 1995-96, 0.9% in 1999, 1.2% in 2002 and 1.8% in 2007-08 |
| Mukinda *et al.* [224] | Cape Winelands Overberg district, Western Cape Province, South Africa; WHO African region | Retrospective case control study (laboratory and hospital data) comparing RMR-TB with HMR-TB | 2004-08 | 91 RMR-TB and 114 HMR-TB | Increase; estimated doubling time of RMR-TB was 2.08, (95%CI 1.7-2.7) years for Western Cape Province and 1.63 (95%CI 1.2-2.7) years for Cape Winelands-Overberg region |
| Seddon *et al.* [225] | Cape Town, Western Cape Province, South Africa; WHO African region | Prospective, single hospital-based survey among children (aged 0-13 years) compared to previous surveys | 2007-09 (compared to 1994-98, 2003-05 & 2005-07) | 4 RMR-TB (1.4%) among 292 TB (2007-09) | Increase; 0% RMR-TB among TB in 1994-98 and 2003-05, 0.7% in 2005-07 and 1.4% in 2007-09 (p=0.009) |

| van Halsema *et al.* [226] | Gauteng Province, South Africa; WHO African region | Retrospective analysis of routine data from 2 gold-mining companies | 2002-08 | 27 RMR-TB (1.3%) among 2007 TB in company A and 1 (0.07%) RMR-TB among 1472 TB in company B | Increase; in company A, RMR-TB case notification rate 17.1/100000 in 2002 and 55.3/100000 in 2008 (p<0.001); No change in company B |
|---|---|---|---|---|---|
| ***Low HIV prevalence countries*** | | | | | |
| He *et al.* [227] | Shandong Province, China; WHO Western Pacific region | Retrospective analysis of surveillance data | 2007-14 | 298 RMR-TB (2.2%) among 13486 TB | Increase; RMR-TB among TB increasing at 0.1% annually (p=0.003) |
| Kruijshaar *et al.* [228] | England, Wales, Northern Ireland, United Kingdom; WHO European region | Retrospective analysis of surveillance data | 1998-2005 | 92 RMR-TB (0.3%) among 28485 TB | No trend; RMR-TB among TB varied from 0.1% to 0.5% annually |
| Lan *et al.* [229] | Guizhou Province, China; WHO Western Pacific region | Prospective, hospital-based cohort study, compared to previous studies | 2013-15 (compared to previous studies in 2008-10 and 2011-12 | 11 RMR-TB (2.4%) among 462 TB | Decrease; RMR-TB among TB declined from 6.5% in the periods 2008-10 and 2011-12 to 2.4% in 2013-15 |
| Prach *et al.* [230] | California, USA; WHO/PAHO region of the Americans | Retrospective analysis of surveillance data matched with HIV registry data | 1993-2008 | 178 RMR-TB (0.4%) among 42582 TB | Decrease; RMR-TB among RR-TB declined from 31% (95%CI 26-38%) in 1993-96 to 11% (5-19%) in 2005-08 (p<0.001); 13% annual decline among HIV positive compared to 6% in HIV negative |
| Tao *et al.* [231] | Shandong Province, China; WHO Western Pacific region | Retrospective analysis of surveillance data (rural populations) | 2006-15 | 163 RMR-TB (1.7%) among 9572 TB | Increase; 9.3% annual increase among treatment naïve TB (p=0.03) and 14% among previously treated (p=0.004) |
| Wang *et al.* [232] | Taipei, Taiwan; WHO Western Pacific region | Retrospective hospital-based cohort study | 1996-99 | 45 RMR-TB (9.9%) among 453 TB | No trend; RMR-TB ranged from 5.9% to 13.9% annually |

**Abbreviations:** RR-TB = Rifampicin-resistant Tuberculosis; RMR-TB = Rifampicin Mono-Resistant Tuberculosis; HMR-TB = Isoniazid Mono-Resistant Tuberculosis; HIV = Human Immunodeficiency Virus; KZN = KwaZulu-Natal; USA = United States of America; UNAIDS = Joint United Nations Programme on HIV/AIDS; CI = Confidence interval; WHO = World Health Organization; PAHO = Pan American Health Organization
**Definitions:** *High HIV prevalence countries* = A high proportion of estimated country/regional adult (15-49 years) HIV prevalence in 2018, according to data provided by UNAIDS. *Low HIV prevalence countries* = A low proportion of estimated country/regional adult (15-49 years) HIV prevalence in 2018, according to data provided by UNAIDS.

<u>**Table 4. 3**</u> Transmission of RMR-TB found in 6/25 (24%) eligible studies

| **Reference** | **Country & Region** | **Type of Study** | **Study period** | **Sample size** | **Method for assessing transmission** | **Transmission (summary)** |
|---|---|---|---|---|---|---|
| ***High HIV prevalence countries*** | | | | | | |
| Dramowski *et al.* [222] | Cape Town, Western Cape Province, South Africa; WHO African region | Prospective, hospital-based description of childhood RMR-TB | 2003-09 | 18 children with RMR-TB | Known contact with adult index cases | 5/18 children with RMR-TB exposed to adult RMR-TB cases, suggesting primary transmission |
| Mukinda *et al.* [224] | Cape Winelands Overberg district, Western Cape Province, South Africa; WHO African region | Retrospective case control study (laboratory and hospital data) comparing RMR-TB with HMR-TB | 2004-08 | 91 RMR-TB and 114 HMR-TB | Spoligotyping and sequencing of the *rpoB* gene | Confirmed RMR-TB transmission in 12/91 cases (13.5%) |
| ***Low HIV prevalence countries*** | | | | | | |
| Lutfey *et al.* [48] | New York City, USA; WHO/PAHO region of the Americans | Case series | 1992 | 26 RMR-TB strains from 20 patients | IS*6110* RFLP fingerprinting and sequencing of the *rpoB* gene | No genetic links between patients |
| Ridzon *et al.* [233] | 11 study sites across USA; WHO/PAHO region of the Americans | Multicentre matched case control study comparing RMR-TB with DS-TB | 1993-95 | 77 RMR-TB cases (3 were lab contaminants and 10 had an identified epidemiological link to another case with RMR-TB – excluded from analysis); | Contact investigation data; IS*6110* RFLP fingerprinting and sequencing of the *rpoB* gene | Of the 77 RMR-TB cases (excluding 3 lab contaminants), 10/74 (14%) were estimated to be due to recent transmission |

|  |  |  |  | Thus, a total of 64 RMR-TB cases and 126 DS-TB controls |  |  |
|---|---|---|---|---|---|---|
| Sheen *et al.* [234] | Lima, Peru; WHO/PAHO region of the Americans | Retrospective analysis of stored TB strains from research studies | 1999-2005 | 37 RMR-TB (4.7%) among 794 TB | Spoligotyping to detect closely related clusters | RMR-TB not associated with clustering compared to DS-TB (aOR 0.43, 0.2-0.9) |
| Velayati *et al.* [235] | Iran; WHO Eastern Mediterranean region | Prospective study of TB patients remaining or becoming sputum smear positive during treatment | 2010-11 | 92 RMR-TB (7.4%) among 1242 TB | Spoligotyping, MIRU-VNTR and epidemiological data | 68% of 92 RMR-TB isolates were clustered genotypically. Epidemiological links in 7 (13%) |

**Abbreviations:** DS-TB = Drug-susceptible Tuberculosis; RMR-TB = Rifampicin Mono-Resistant Tuberculosis; HMR-TB = Isoniazid Mono-Resistant Tuberculosis; IS*6110* RFLP = IS*6110* Restriction Fragment Length Polymorphism (RFLP) Fingerprinting; MIRU-VNTR = Mycobacterium interspersed repetitive unit-variable number tandem repeat; lab = laboratory; USA = United States of America; UNAIDS = Joint United Nations Programme on HIV/AIDS; WHO = World Health Organization; PAHO = Pan American Health Organization
**Definitions:** *High HIV prevalence countries* = A high proportion of estimated country/regional adult (15-49 years) HIV prevalence in 2018, according to data provided by UNAIDS. *Low HIV prevalence countries* = A low proportion of estimated country/regional adult (15-49 years) HIV prevalence in 2018, according to data provided by UNAIDS.

Table 4. 4 Risk factors for RMR-TB found in 14/25 (56%) eligible studies

| Reference | Country & Region | Type of Study & risk factors assessed | Study period | Sample size | Risk factors for RMR-TB (HIV related) | Risk factors for RMR-TB (other) |
|---|---|---|---|---|---|---|
| ***High HIV prevalence countries*** | | | | | | |
| Coovadia *et al.* [89] | Durban, KZN Province, South Africa; WHO African region | Retrospective analysis of laboratory data (logistic regression assessing whether gender and age group were risk factors for RMR-TB) | 2007-09 | 1 466 RMR-TB (8.8%) among 16748 RR-TB | HIV status not reported | RMR-TB among males (OR 1.42, 93%CI 1.27-1.60) compared to females<br>Age 25-29 increased RMR-TB over time (compared to aged 50+) |
| Mukinda *et al.* [224] | Cape Winelands Overberg district, Western Cape Province, South Africa; WHO African region | Retrospective case control study (laboratory and hospital data) comparing RMR-TB with HMR-TB (logistic regression with inclusion of variables significant on univariate analysis) | 2007-09 | 91 RMR-TB and 114 HMR-TB | ART before DR-TB treatment start (aOR 6.4, 1.3-31.8) were identified as a significant risk factor for RMR-TB compared to HMR-TB | Age ≥ 40 (aOR 5.8, 95%CI 2.4-13.6), alcohol use (aOR 4.8, 2.0-11.3), sputum smear negativity (aOR 3.0, 1.4-5.0) and more recent diagnosis (aOR 4.0, 1.8-8.9) were identified as significant risk factors for RMR-TB compared to HMR-TB |
| van Helsema *et al.* [226] | Gauteng Province, South Africa; WHO African region | Retrospective analysis of routine data from gold-mining companies with comparison of prevalence ratios by previous TB treatment and HIV | 2002-08 | 27 RMR-TB (1.1%) among 2422 TB patients (with available DST) | Prevalence ratio for RMR-TB by HIV status not reported | Previous TB treatment (prev ratio 6.1, 95% CI2.6-14.4) |
| ***Low HIV prevalence countries*** | | | | | | |
| LoBue *et al.* [236] | San Diego County, USA; WHO/PAHO region of the Americans | Retrospective analysis of surveillance data (logistic regression with inclusion of variables significant | 1993-2002 | 11 RMR-TB (0.4%) among 2883 TB | HIV positivity (aOR 5.6, 95% CI 1.6-19.4) | Previous TB treatment (aOR 3.9, 95% CI 0.8-18.5) |

| | | on univariate analysis) | | | | |
|---|---|---|---|---|---|---|
| Moore *et al.* [237] | USA; WHO/PAHO region of the Americans | Retrospective analysis of national surveillance data (comparison of RMR-TB prevalence by HIV status) | 1993-96 | 67340 TB (with drug susceptibility testing) | RMR-TB higher among HIV positive individuals (2.6% versus 0.2%) (HIV status known for 46% of participants aged 25-44) | No other risk factors assessed |
| Munsiff *et al.* [238] | New York City, USA; WHO/PAHO region of the Americans | Case control study assessing the emergence of acquired rifampicin resistance among HIV positive patients during treatment | 1993-94 | 29 acquired RR-TB and 58 DS-TB | HIV positivity (aOR 5.6, 1.7-18.6) | Poor adherence (aOR 11.0, 3.3-37.3), sputum smear positivity (aOR 4.1, 1.2-13.2) |
| Prach *et al.* [230] | California, USA; WHO/PAHO region of the Americans | Retrospective analysis of surveillance data matched with HIV registry data (comparison of prevalence ratios between RMR-TB and DS-TB) | 1993-2008 | 178 RMR-TB (0.4%) among 42582 TB | HIV positivity (prev ratio 7.2, 95%CI 5.2-10.0). Among HIV positive, previous TB diagnosis (prev ratio 3.1, 1.5-6.3) and male sex (prev ratio 1.5, 1.1-2.1) | Previous TB diagnosis (prev ratio 2.8, 1.8-4.3) |
| Ridzon *et al.* [233] | 11 study sites across USA; WHO/PAHO region of the Americans | Multicentre matched case control study comparing RMR-TB with DS-TB (logistic regression) | 1993-95 | 64 RMR-TB and 126 DS-TB | Among HIV positive, prior antifungal therapy (aOR 4.7, p<0.01), diarrhoea (aOR 3.0, p=0.05), rifabutin use (aOR undefined, p<0.001). Among HIV positive without rifabutin use, prior ART (aOR 4.7, p=0.01). Among HIV positive with rifabutin use, diarrhoea (aOR undefined, p<0.01) | Overall, previous TB treatment (OR 3.0, 1.1-7.9) |
| Robert *et al.* [239] | France; WHO European region | Retrospective analysis of hospital | 1995-97 | 12 RMR-TB (0.5%) among | HIV positivity (aOR 27.2, 95%CI 7.2-102.6) | Previous TB treatment (aOR 10.9, 3.4-35.3) |

| | | | | | | |
|---|---|---|---|---|---|---|
| | | surveillance data (logistic regression comparing RMR-TB with all other TB) | | 2601 TB | | |
| Sandman *et al.* [240] | New York City, USA; WHO/PAHO region of the Americans | Retrospective hospital-based case-control study comparing RMR-TB with DS-TB | 1990-97 | 21 RMR-TB and 48 DS-TB | HIV positivity (OR 10.9, 1.1-undefined). Among HIV positive, extrapulmonary TB (OR 2.9, 1.0-8.1) & prior opportunistic infections (OR 8.3, 1.5-44.7) | Previous TB episode (OR 7, 95%CI 2-24). Among treatment naive patients, prison exposure (OR 8.7, 1.2-63.2). |
| Sheen *et al.* [234] | Lima, Peru; WHO/PAHO region of the Americans | Retrospective analysis of stored TB strains from research studies (comparison between RMR-TB and DS-TB) | 1999-2005 | 37 RMR-TB (4.7%) among 794 TB | HIV positivity not significant (aOR 1.7, 95% CI 0.8-3.5) | No risk factors significant |
| Smith *et al.* [219] | Up to 81 countries & subnational settings | Retrospective analysis of routine data reported to WHO (comparison of RMR-TB by categories of MDR-TB prevalence) | Reports from 1997, 2000, 2004, 2008 | 1615 RMR-TB (0.7%) among 221084 TB (12.9% RMR-TB among RR-TB) | HIV status not assessed | Increased RMR-TB prevalence associated with decreased MDR-TB prevalence. Low MDR-TB prevalence (<1.5%) 26.5% RMR-TB among RR-TB, Medium MDR-TB prevalence (1.5-4.6%) 19.2% RMR-TB among RR-TB, High MDR-TB prevalence (>4.6%) 9.8% RMR-TB among RR-TB |
| Vernon *et al.* [241] | USA and Canada; WHO/PAHO region of the Americans | Analysis of clinical trial data assessing relapse with RMR-TB among HIV positive TB patients | 1995-97 | 61 HIV positive TB patients receiving once or twice weekly TB treatment | 4 RMR-TB in once weekly group compared to none in twice weekly groups (p=0.05). Among once weekly group, RMR-TB relapse associated with low CD4 (p=0.02) and use of antifungal treatment (p=0.04) | Patients who relapsed with RMR-TB were younger (median age 29 vs 41 years), had extrapulmonary TB (75% vs 18% p=0.03) and antifungal treatment (75% vs 9%, p=0.006) |
| Villegas *et al.* [242] | Lima, Peru; WHO/PAHO region of the Americans | Prospective observational cohort study among treatment naive smear positive TB (logistic regression | 2010-11 | 24 RMR-TB (2.3%) among 1039 TB | HIV positivity (aOR=9.4, 95% CI 1.9-47.8) | No risk factors significant |

| | | comparing RMR-TB to DS-TB) | | | | |
|---|---|---|---|---|---|---|

**Abbreviations:** ART = Antiretroviral treatment; DS-TB = Drug susceptible Tuberculosis; RR-TB = Rifampicin resistant Tuberculosis; RMR-TB = Rifampicin Mono-Resistant Tuberculosis; HMR-TB = Isoniazid Mono-Resistant Tuberculosis; HIV = Human Immunodeficiency Virus infection; DST = Drug susceptibility testing; IS*6110* RFLP = IS*6110* Restriction Fragment Length Polymorphism (RFLP) Fingerprinting; MIRU-VNTR = Mycobacterium interspersed repetitive unit-variable number tandem repeat; KZN = KwaZulu-Natal; USA = United States of America; UNAIDS = Joint United Nations Programme on HIV/AIDS; CI = Confidence interval; OR = Odds ratio; prev ratio = prevalence ratio; WHO = World Health Organization; PAHO = Pan American Health Organization

**Definitions:** *High HIV prevalence countries* = A high proportion of estimated country/regional adult (15-49 years) HIV prevalence in 2018, according to data provided by UNAIDS. *Low HIV prevalence countries* = A low proportion of estimated country/regional adult (15-49 years) HIV prevalence in 2018, according to data provided by UNAIDS.

### 4.3.2 Temporal trends of RMR-TB

For temporal trends of RMR-TB, 13 eligible studies were included (Table 4.2). Studies were carried out between 1996-2015, and included data from four WHO regions including the African region (7), the Western pacific region (4), the WHO/PAHO (Pan American Health Organization) region of the Americas (1), and the European region (1). African countries consisted of six studies from South Africa and one from Botswana. Countries from the Western pacific region included China (3) and Taiwan (1). American and European studies were from California, United States of America (USA) and the United Kingdom, respectively.

Among the seven studies reporting temporal trends in high HIV prevalence settings, six were from South Africa and one from Botswana. Five of the six studies in South Africa suggested an increasing trend over time, with one of these studies reporting an increase in one of the two settings assessed, but not the other [226]. The majority of these studies described RMR-TB either in terms of absolute numbers, or as a proportion of all TB. No temporal trend was observed in a large study assessing RMR-TB among RR-TB from one South African province; however, only three years of data were included [89]. Also, no change was observed over time from the study in Botswana (two years of data) [223].

Among the six studies from low HIV prevalence countries, two showed increasing trends for RMR-TB among all TB over time, both studies were from the same province in China. [227, 231]. Another study from China showed declining RMR-TB among TB [229]. Decreasing RMR-TB among all TB was also observed in a study from California, USA [230], while no trend was observed in the UK [228]. The final study from Taiwan also showed no trend over time, although the time period assessed was relatively narrow (1996-1999) [232].

### 4.3.3 Transmission of RMR-TB

For transmission of RMR-TB, only six eligible studies were included (Table 4.3). Studies were conducted between 1992-2011, from the WHO African region (2/6), the WHO/PAHO region of the Americas (3/6), and the Eastern Mediterranean region (1/6).

All high HIV prevalence studies were from the Western Cape Province, South Africa (2/6) [222, 224]. Transmission was assessed among children with known contact with adult index cases, and studies among adults included methods such as spoligotyping and sequencing of the *rpoB* gene. All low HIV prevalence countries were from America and Iran (4/6) [48, 233-235]. Additional methods of transmission assessment included utilising epidemiological data to assess transmission links between patients, IS*6110* RFLP fingerprinting and MIRU-VNTR typing. The highest percentage of confirmed RMR-TB transmission was found at 13% (in South Africa and Iran) and 14% (across USA) [224, 233, 235].

### 4.3.4 Risk factors of RMR-TB

There were 14 articles that assessed risk factors for RMR-TB (Table 4.4). Studies were carried out between 1990 and 2011. High HIV prevalence countries were all from South Africa (3/14), whereas low HIV prevalence countries were from the United States (9/14) and Europe (1/14). The remaining study included data from 81 countries and subnational settings. This latter study reported that increased RMR-TB prevalence (>40% RR-TB isolates among new TB cases) was associated with relatively lower MDR-TB prevalence (among all TB) (one third of all countries and subnational settings) as detected by GeneXpert MTB/RIF (Xpert). The authors suggest confirming Xpert results with conventional DST with confirmation of INH susceptibility testing [219].

#### *High HIV prevalence countries*

- ***HIV and other risk factors***

Among the three studies from South Africa, Mukinda *et al.* [224] was the only study that showed significant risk factors for RMR-TB compared to HMR-TB; these included previous use of antiretroviral therapy among adult patients with advanced HIV disease, alcohol abuse, sputum smear negativity and recent DR-TB diagnosis. Their study also reported increased RMR-TB compared to HMR-TB among HIV positive individuals in the age group ≥40 years (OR 5.8, 95%CI 2.4-13.6) compared to those aged <40 [224]. On the contrary, Coovadia *et al.* [89] found an increase of RMR-TB among RR-TB over time among the age group 25 to 29 years (p=0.009), when compared to the age group over 50 years. Furthermore, the study found that males had 42% increased odds of RMR-TB (among all RR-TB) compared to females during the years 2007-2009, after adjusting for time and age (OR 1.42; 93% CI 1.27-1.60; p<0.0001). Unfortunately, HIV status was not reported. Lastly, previous TB treatment was a significant risk factor for RMR-TB compared to all TB, in South African gold mines [226]. However, HIV status was also not reported in the study.

#### *Low HIV prevalence countries*

- ***HIV as a risk factor***

RMR-TB among either RR-TB [238], or among all TB cases [237, 242] was found to be significantly associated with HIV positive individuals with no history of previous TB treatment in two studies from the USA [237, 238] and one study from Peru [242]. However, another study from Peru found that HIV positivity was not significant [234]. Other RMR-TB risk factors among HIV positive individuals included poor adherence during prior TB treatment and sputum smear positivity [238].

- ***HIV, previous TB treatment and other risk factors***

RMR-TB among all TB cases was found to be significantly associated with a history of previous TB treatment among individuals who were HIV positive (at RR-TB diagnosis) in low HIV prevalence countries such as Europe [239] and several studies from the USA [230, 233, 236, 240, 241].

A number of risk factors for RMR-TB were found among HIV positive individuals with TB and previous treatment history. Risk factors found among this group of individuals that were independently associated with RMR-TB were prior rifabutin use [233], antifungal therapy [233, 241], and diarrhoea (presumed malabsorption of TB drugs) with rifabutin use [233]. However, in HIV positive individuals without prior rifabutin use, prior antiretroviral treatment (ART) was also a significant risk factor for RMR-TB. Evidence also suggested that among HIV positive patients who relapsed with RMR-TB, risk factors included severe immunosuppression with lower baseline CD4 counts (at the time of relapse) in a study from North America [241]. For gender related risk factors, Prach *et al.* [230] found a higher prevalence of RMR-TB among all TB cases among males. This was in agreement with the South African study by Coovadia *et al.* [89]. For age related risk factors, a North American study by Vernon *et al.* [241] found that previously treated patients who relapsed with RMR-TB were younger (median age 29 vs 41 years) compared to those who relapsed with drug-susceptible TB (DS-TB). Thus, the study by Vernon *et al.* [241], corresponded well with the study by Coovadia *et al.* [89], where RMR-TB among RR-TB was more likely to occur in the age group 25-29 years compared to >50 years. Lastly among individuals with HIV-TB co-infection and previous TB treatment, other reports demonstrated a significant association of RMR-TB with extrapulmonary TB [240, 241] and prior opportunistic infections (not clearly specified) [240]. There was also an association between RMR-TB and prison exposure among treatment naïve TB patients from the same study [240].

## 4.4 Discussion

There are a wide range of factors that may contribute to the high and often varied burden of RMR-TB within various geographical settings. Hence, we assessed RMR-TB data related to temporal trends, transmission and risk factors. Overall, these findings clearly show the paucity of studies specifically addressing RMR-TB, with many studies conducted decades ago.

Recent data from the WHO global TB report of 2019, showed a broad range of RMR-TB prevalence among all RR-TB among the 30 high MDR/RR-TB burden countries globally [2]. In 2018, RMR-TB percentages among all RR-TB ranged from 0% in certain geographical areas in Europe (Belarus), Asia (Myanmar, Kyrgyzstan) and East Africa (Ethiopia); to >38% in East and South Africa (Somalia - 39%; South Africa and Kenya - 38%), Central Asia (Uzbekisan - 43%, and Kazakhstan - 41%); with the highest percentage of RMR-TB found in Central Africa (DR Congo - 45%) [2]. The underlying questions are whether these differences could be influenced by variation in the propensity of different TB strain lineages to develop RIF R, and be subsequently transmitted; genetic differences in the population being treated for TB (through varying pharmacokinetics, resulting in differing risk of RIF R acquisition during TB treatment); or due to an association with HIV and varied HIV prevalence in different settings [33]. Previous studies found that the diversity of TB strains; for instance different strain lineages; varied in their capacity to transmit, resulting in the intensity of an individuals immune response and TB disease severity [243, 244]. These diverse TB strains may also have varying propensities for developing RIF R [245-247]. Nonetheless, this field of research requires further investigation and elucidation.

Within the nine provinces of South Africa, considerable variation in the increase of RMR-TB over time among either RR-TB, or among all TB was found [4, 222, 224-226]. This was supported by data from China where an increase in trends were seen in one province (Shandong), but not the other (Guizhou). Furthermore, the findings from this review highlight that not only high HIV prevalence countries (like South Africa), but also low HIV prevalence countries (like China), report increasing trends of RMR-TB across countries within specific provinces. There is still uncertainty as to why there is a significant increase of RMR-TB observed over time in some geographical settings and not in others, regardless of high/low HIV prevalence within a setting. In this systematic review, most of the data from high HIV prevalence settings came from South Africa.

A dynamic transmission model providing data from six countries from different geographical settings, showed that most incident MDR-TB from majority of high MDR-TB burden settings was due to transmission rather than acquisition [8]. Whether this is the same for RMR-TB is unknown. Nonetheless, the results from this systematic review clearly show that RMR-TB transmission occurs in both high and low HIV prevalence countries, even though data is scarce.

Additionally, these review findings revealed that HIV positivity was significantly associated with RMR-TB among both RR-TB and all TB, regardless of individuals that had previous TB treatment history or not. Thus, these findings suggest that both transmission and acquisition are important contributing factors for RMR-TB, with varied risk factors found in different geographical settings. However, knowledge on the factors that may be contributing to MDR- and RMR-TB transmission and/or acquisition in HIV endemic regions, is lacking [67].

In the past, two systematic reviews focused on the association between HIV and MDR-TB among new and previously treated patients [248, 249]. Both reviews found increased risks of MDR-TB among new, TB treatment naïve patients compared to previously treated patients, suggesting a stronger association of HIV with transmission rather than acquisition. This may be due to nosocomial transmission, specifically in high HIV prevalence settings, where there is higher exposure of MDR-TB together with increased HIV immunosuppression that coincide within healthcare facilities [67]. Additionally, the authors suggest that the risk of transmission increases in other congregate settings [67]. Whether these study findings for MDR-TB is the same for RMR-TB, is yet unknown.

On the other hand, another systematic review suggested that HIV infection was specifically associated with increased risk of RIF R acquisition, compared to HIV negative individuals [37]. Evidence of RMR-TB associated with advanced HIV disease with low CD4 counts; particularly among patients receiving ART prior to TB diagnosis, was reported [241]. Studies also suggest that drug malabsorption may result from gut infection with opportunistic pathogens or HIV enteropathy that may result in low serum levels of the drug, followed by selection of RMR-TB mutants [48, 49, 240, 250]. Moreover, drug to drug interactions among TB patients who are HIV positive, receiving multiple medications, can alter the pharmacokinetics of anti-TB medications [240, 251]. Notably, reports of drug to drug interactions between RIF and antifungal drugs, such as co-trimoxazole or the azole group have shown an increase in half-life of RIF [49, 241, 252-254]. However, these factors appear to be multifactorial and driven by unknown mechanisms.

Additionally, systematic reviews on the risk factors for MDR-TB showed variation across different settings. These reviews indicated that previous TB treatment and HIV were key risk factors across different settings [255, 256]. RMR-TB risk factors from this systematic review (within this book) indicate that HIV and RMR-TB co-infection are associated with shared risk factors such as younger age, male gender, alcohol use, prison exposure, and extrapulmonary TB. RMR-TB was more likely to occur among younger age groups in some studies [89, 241]. Nonetheless, many studies used different cut-off points for age groups, and the association between age and risk of RMR-TB is not well defined. For instance, Law *et al.* [257] suggests that age related differences in TB treatment adherence could be possible, as elderly patients lead a more sedentary lifestyle post-retirement suggesting relatively good TB treatment adherence. In contrast, this study also suggests that younger patients who often work, study, travel or are involved in various daily activities, are more likely to have acquired resistance compared to the elderly [257]. Some studies in this review have also shown that the male gender were more likely to develop RMR-TB than females [89, 230]. Similarly, MDR-TB among all TB cases were more likely to be male (compared to female) and younger than 65 years (compared to >65 years), in a review by Faustini *et al.* [255]. These differences could be due to gender dissimilarities of access to health-care facilities or exposure to other risk factors such as the misuse of alcohol. Studies also suggest that this association may be due to socio-economic factors and poor knowledge regarding the importance of TB treatment adherence [258].

There is evidence that individuals who misuse alcohol are less likely to complete their full course of TB treatment [259]. This association, together with poor adherence by individuals from unstable social backgrounds, may lead to the selection of resistant mutants during treatment [259-261]. Extrapulmonary TB (EPTB) was also reported as a risk factor for RMR-TB in two papers identified within this book systematic review [240, 241]. It is highly possible that EPTB among HIV infected individuals may lead to the development of RR-TB with a combination of the following: advanced immunosuppression, complex interactions within the cellular immune system, and a higher total bacterial burden. Another possibility could be that TB drugs are distributed at different concentrations to extrapulmonary compartments, resulting in the development of RMR-TB [240]. Lastly, in this review chapter within this book, prison exposure among treatment naïve patients was another risk factor for RMR-TB patients who were HIV positive [230, 240]. This could be linked to many shared risk factors for RMR-TB, including HIV together with malnutrition causing poor immunity, overcrowding, poor access to diagnosis and treatment; resulting in manifestation of transmission rates within prisons.

A limitation of this review was the scarcity of data related to RMR-TB, that may not be a true reflection of findings in all countries worldwide. Nonetheless, this review contributed to increasing the overall knowledge of RMR-TB temporal trends, transmission and risk factors; and follow-up studies could be conducted to better understand these associations.

## 4.5 Conclusion

This systematic review reveals that the epidemiology of RMR-TB varies significantly across different settings all over the world and constitutes a large proportion of the RR-TB burden worldwide. Factors that weaken the immune system (for instance HIV, smoking, alcohol abuse, use of drugs with immunosuppressant properties) may all be risk factors for developing RR-TB. Variation of pharmacokinetic effects among RR-TB individuals (especially among those who are HIV positive) may have increasing effects in combination with any of the risk factors described to be associated with RMR-TB.

Even though RMR-TB emerged through selection of RIF R during treatment, transmission of these strains could increase if overlooked. However, evidence on the transmission of RMR-TB is limited in this review, with reports of RMR-TB transmission links in three clusters and epidemiological associations. These results suggest that RMR-TB may have a lower tendency to transmit than for MDR-TB as reported by one of the studies in this review.

Furthermore, next generation- or whole genome sequencing could eventually give better insight on RMR-TB transmission than previously used methods reported in this review. There has also been no clinical trials and few observational data designed to optimise the treatment of patients with RMR-TB, especially among HIV and TB co-infected individuals. In general, studies related to this field of research are ill-defined and need further comprehension.

# CHAPTER FIVE

# 5. Epidemiology of rifampicin mono-resistant TB in Khayelitsha

**The risk of RMR-TB relative to MDR-TB among RR-TB patients in Khayelitsha: Impact of HIV infection during previous TB treatment**

## 5.1 Introduction

In 2018, the World Health Organization (WHO) reported that an estimated 10 million individuals developed *Mycobacterium tuberculosis (M.tb)* disease, a number that has remained relatively stable during the recent years (2015-2018). Moreover, in 2018, global mortality due to *M.tb* was an estimated 1.2 million among HIV negative individuals and 251 000 among HIV positive individuals [2]. Whilst transmission has accentuated the spread of the rifampicin-resistant TB (RR-TB) epidemic, a better understanding of the factors contributing to the acquisition of resistance is vital. Rifampicin resistance (RIF R) acquisition is the evolution of mutations conferring drug resistance under drug pressure during TB treatment. Worldwide and within South Africa, the WHO estimated that 3.4% of new TB cases had MDR/RR-TB in 2018. Additionally, MDR/RR-TB among previously TB treated cases was an estimated 18% globally and 7.1% in South Africa during 2018 [2]. Furthermore, HIV-TB co-infected individuals constituted an estimated 11% and 59% globally and within South Africa, respectively. Approximately 87% (globally and within South Africa) of HIV-TB co-infected individuals were receiving antiretroviral therapy (ART) at the time of TB diagnosis [2].

Moreover, a previous systematic review and meta-analysis found that HIV-TB co-infection was significantly associated with an increased risk of TB drug resistance acquisition [37]. Another study reported that rifampicin mono-resistant TB (RMR-TB) was associated with advanced HIV disease in patients with low CD4 counts; particularly among those receiving ART prior to TB diagnosis [241]. In addition, the systematic review within this book (Chapter 4) describes significant associations between RMR-TB and HIV positivity among individuals with known history of previous TB treatment in a number of studies [224, 230, 233, 236, 239, 240].

Throughout the nine provinces of South Africa, considerable variation was found in the proportion of RMR-TB among all RR-TB according to the South African national drug-resistant TB (DR-TB) survey results of 2012-2014 [4, 5]. Previously, the main driver of DR-TB was considered to be the acquisition of drug resistance during patient treatment. However, studies now show that the fitness of DR-TB is diverse and that most multi-drug resistant TB (MDR-TB) cases are in fact due to transmission rather than due to resistance acquisition during TB treatment [8, 10]. Yet, in the setting of Khayelitsha, we do not know if the same applies for RMR-TB and whether acquired drug resistance is still a major contributor.

Within this book (Chapter 4, systematic review) , evidence does suggest an association between HIV and RIF R acquisition. Thus, the study objectives within this chapter of the book are firstly to describe the overall prevalence of RMR-TB among RR-TB patients diagnosed in Khayelitsha (a high HIV-TB prevalence setting) over a 10 year period (2008-2017 inclusive); and to secondly assess the relative risk of RMR-TB versus MDR-TB among RR-TB patients diagnosed in Khayelitsha over a 3 year period (2013-2015 inclusive), by HIV and ART status during previous TB treatment. The hypothesis is that HIV infection during first-line TB treatment is associated with a greater risk of subsequent RMR-TB relative to MDR-TB in Khayelitsha.

## 5.2 Methods

### 5.2.1 Study population: Prevalence during 2008 to 2017

All patients diagnosed with bacteriologically confirmed RR-TB across a 10 year period (2008-2017) in Khayelitsha were included. Patients who were only diagnosed with GeneXpert MTB/RIF (Xpert) without subsequent DST for determination of isoniazid resistance were excluded, as were those who had second-line TB treatment previously.

### 5.2.2 Study population: Cohort during 2013 to 2015

All patients diagnosed with bacteriologically confirmed RR-TB across 2013-2015 were included. As before, patients who were only diagnosed with Xpert without subsequent DST were excluded, as were those who had second-line TB treatment previously. Limited data was available on previous TB treatment regimens and TB treatment outcomes of patients within this cohort.

### 5.2.3 Additional data collection for cohort

While current HIV status, i.e. at the time of RR-TB treatment, and previous TB treatment status were routinely recorded on the Médecins sans Frontières (MSF) DR-TB database, whether patients were HIV positive and receiving ART during previous TB treatment episodes was not recorded. In order to obtain this information, data from the Public Health Data Centre (PHDC) in the Western Cape were accessed [197].

The PHDC [a health information exchange] was established in 2015, to draw together data from: specific disease monitoring systems (e.g. for TB, HIV), laboratory and pharmacy supply data, hospital and primary care registration systems, and population registers. While the PHDC primarily aims to directly support patient care, the data environment also allows epidemiological analyses to be conducted, in a manner that does not compromise patient confidentiality. To access data, a list of patient-level identifiers was submitted to the PHDC. PHDC staff then accessed data related to HIV testing and treatment, along with all TB episodes connected to each individual. Both HIV and TB data were drawn from specific disease registers, pharmaceutical supply data, laboratory data, and hospital admission data.

### 5.2.4 Data analysis of cohort

Firstly, we determined whether patients had received any prior TB treatment (Figure 5.1). This was done by drawing on the routinely collected data from the MSF database and data supplied from the PHDC. For patients with no record of previous TB treatment, patients were classified as either HIV negative or positive at RR-TB diagnosis. For previously TB treated patients we then determined HIV status during previous TB treatment. Patients who were HIV negative at RR-TB diagnosis were classified as HIV negative during previous TB treatment. For those who were HIV positive and had previous TB treatment, PHDC data were used to determine the date that the patient was first known to be HIV positive. This included data from enrolment into HIV care, CD4 laboratory testing, and initiation of ART. PHDC data was also used to determine dates of all previous TB treatment episodes. Any patient who had at least one TB treatment episode, defined as registration in the TB treatment register or supply of first-line TB drugs, after they were known to be HIV positive, was classified as HIV positive during previous TB treatment. Patients who were HIV positive at the time of RR-TB diagnosis, and had previous TB treatment, but for whom the date first known to be HIV positive could not be determined, were classified separately. HIV positive patients who were known to have HIV during previous TB treatment were classified as being on ART during previous TB treatment if an ART start date was before any previous TB treatment episode (Figure 5.1).

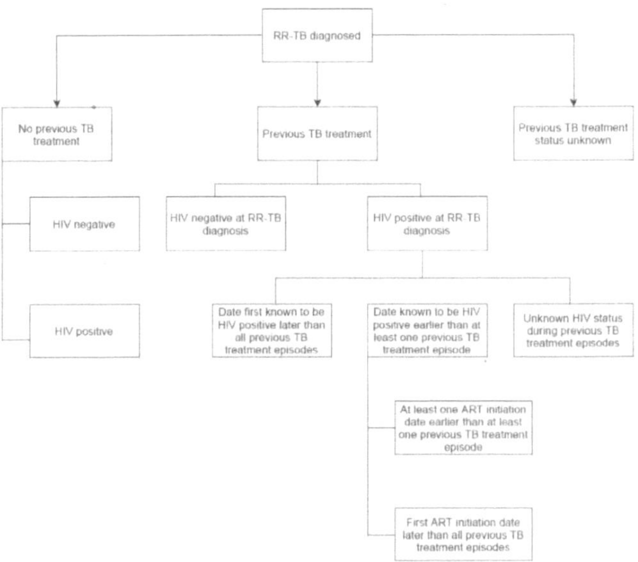


**Figure 5. 1** Diagram representing the analysis of available data

## 5.3 Results

### 5.3.1 Overall prevalence of RR-TB patients in Khayelitsha during 2008 to 2017

Among the 2114 newly diagnosed RR-TB patients between 2008 and 2017, 119 (6%) were excluded as they only had an Xpert RR-TB diagnosis, with no subsequent DST (Table 5.1). Therefore, over the 10 year period, there were 1995 individuals diagnosed with RR-TB in Khayelitsha, of whom 453 (23%) had RMR-TB (Table 5.1). The proportion of RMR-TB among all RR-TB by year ranged from 17-31%, with both the lowest proportion of 17% in 2011 significantly lower than other years ($p<0.05$) and the highest proportion of 31% in 2014 higher than in other years ($p<0.01$).

**Table 5. 1** Total number of routinely diagnosed RR-TB cases by year of diagnosis from 2008-17 in Khayelitsha.

| Year | Total number of RR-TB diagnosed | RMR-TB n (% of total number of RR-TB diagnosed per year) | p-value * |
|---|---|---|---|
| **2008** | 209 | 46 (22%) | *0.80* |
| **2009** | 221 | 48 (22%) | *0.71* |
| **2010** | 212 | 40 (19%) | *0.15* |
| **2011** | 192 | 32 (17%) | *0.03* |
| **2012** | 210 | 49 (23%) | *0.81* |
| **2013** | 195 | 45 (23%) | *0.88* |
| **2014** | 213 | 67 (31%) | *0.001* |
| **2015** | 190 | 38 (20%) | *0.35* |
| **2016** | 198 | 52 (26%) | *0.21* |
| **2017** | 155 | 36 (23%) | *0.86* |
| **Total** | 1995 | 453 (23%) | |

* Chi-squared for difference in proportions per year to assess trends over time

### 5.3.2 Cohort description (2013-2015)

Among the 670 newly diagnosed RR-TB patients between 2013 and 2015, 72 (11%) were excluded as they only had an Xpert RR-TB diagnosis, with no subsequent DST. Among the remaining 598 individual patients, 150 (25%) had RMR-TB. There were no significant differences in gender, age, HIV status or percentage started RR-TB treatment between RMR- and MDR-TB (Table 5.2). There was however a significantly higher proportion of RMR-TB among all RR-TB in 2014 compared to the years 2013 and 2015 ($p<0.01$) (Table 5.2).

**Table 5. 2** Demographic and clinical information among RR-TB patients during 2013-15 in Khayelitsha

| | RMR-TB (n=150) | MDR-TB (n=448) | p-value |
|---|---|---|---|
| Female | 77 (51%) | 227 (51%) | *0.88* |
| Median age (IQR) | 33 (20-46) | 35 (21-49) | *0.09* |
| HIV status known (at RR-TB diagnosis) | 148 (99%) | 441 (98%) | *0.89* |
| HIV positive (% of known) | 117 (79%) | 334 (76%) | *0.40* |
| Initiated second-line TB treatment | 134 (89%) | 409 (91%) | *0.47* |
| Year diagnosed (% by year; row) | | | |
| 2013 | 45 (23%) | 150 (77%) | |
| 2014 | 67 (31%) | 146 (67%) | *<0.01 ** |
| 2015 | 38 (20%) | 152 (80%) | |

*p-value comparisons were for 2014 compared to 2013, and 2014 compared to 2015

### 5.3.3 Previous TB treatment status (2013-2015 cohort)

Based on routinely available data (prior to accessing PHDC data), 247 (41%) patients had not been treated for TB prior to being diagnosed with RR-TB. A further 312 (52%) were recorded as having had previous TB treatment, while data were missing for 39 (7%). After linkage of data to that from the PHDC, an additional 64 patients were identified as having had previous treatment (Table 5.3). This left 15 patients (38%) with unknown previous TB treatment status.

**Table 5. 3** Routine data versus data linked after PHDC in the Western Cape Province, with reference to previous TB treatment status

| | **After linkage with PHDC data** | | | |
|---|---|---|---|---|
| **Routine data** | No previous TB treatment (new) | Previous first-line TB treatment | Unknown previous TB treatment status | **Total** |
| No previous TB treatment (new) | 203 | 44 | 0 | 247 |
| Previous first-line TB treatment | 0 | 312 | 0 | 312 |
| Unknown previous TB treatment status | 4 | 20 | 15 | 39 |
| **Total** | **207** | **376** | **15** | **598** |

Among the 376 patients who were previously treated for TB, the number of prior TB treatment episodes was known for 332 (88%). The majority of patients had one prior episode (202, 60%), while 48 (14%) had three or more prior episodes.

### 5.3.4 HIV and ART status during previous TB treatment (2013-2015 cohort)

After linking the cohort with PHDC data, HIV positivity at RR-TB diagnosis was determined for an additional two patients. Among all patients known to be HIV positive at RR-TB diagnosis, at least one ART initiation date was known for 435 (95%). There is often more than one ART initiation date as there are 'lost to follow-up' patients and upon return to care these patients restart ART treatment. There was no significant difference in the proportion of RMR-TB among all RR-TB by HIV status at the time of RR-TB diagnosis (Table 5.4).

**Table 5. 4** RR-TB patients by HIV status at the time of diagnosis during 2013-15 in Khayelitsha

| | **RMR-TB** | **MDR-TB** | **Total** | **p-value** |
|---|---|---|---|---|
| HIV negative | 29 (22%) | 105 (78%) | 134 | *0.29* |
| HIV positive | 120 (26%) | 339 (74%) | 459 | |
| **Total** | **149 (25%)** | **444 (75%)** | **593** | |

### 5.3.5 RMR-TB by HIV and ART status during previous TB treatment (2013-2015 cohort)

Overall, 536 (90%) of patients could be classified into a category based on previous TB treatment, HIV and ART data (Figure 5.2).

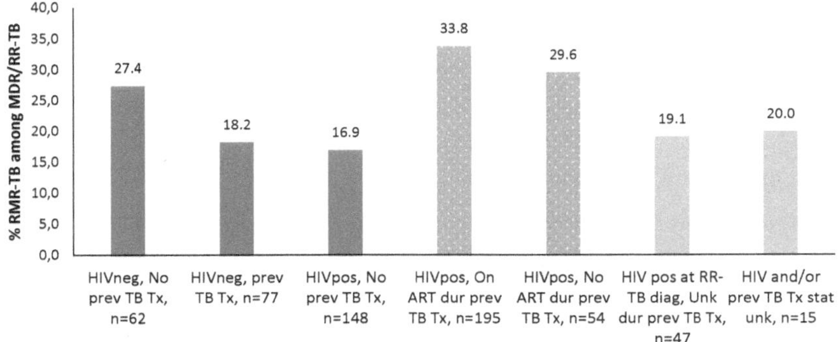


Figure 5. 2 The proportion of RMR-TB among MDR/RR-TB stratified by HIV status, previous TB treatment and ART status

Although numbers are small, there were more RMR-TB among individuals who were HIV positive when they received previous first-line treatment; 33% (82/249) compared to those who were HIV positive at the time of MDR/RR-TB diagnosis and were not previously TB treated; 17% (25/148, p<0.001) and compared to HIV negative individuals with or without previous TB treatment; 22.3% (31/139, p=0.03). There was no significant difference in RMR-TB between HIV positive patients who were on ART and those not on ART during previous TB treatment (p=0.57) (Figure 5.2).

To define the effect size, a Chi-square analysis was conducted (Table 5.5). For simplification, both HIV positive and negative patients with no previous TB treatment were combined, and patients who were HIV positive during previous TB treatment regardless of ART were combined. The odds of RMR-TB versus MDR-TB among patients who were HIV positive during previous TB treatment were twice that for patients with no previous TB treatment; p-value=0.002; OR=2.0 (1.3-3.0). Patients who were HIV negative during previous TB treatment had similar odds of RMR-TB compared to those without previous TB treatment.

**Table 5. 5** Statistical analysis between RMR- and MDR-TB patients by HIV status with or without previous TB treatment

| Category | Odds ratio (95% confidence interval) | p-value |
|---|---|---|
| No previous TB treatment | 1.0 (reference) | |
| HIV positive during previous TB treatment | 2.0 (1.3-3.0) | *0.002* |
| HIV negative during previous TB treatment | 0.89 (0.46-1.7) | *0.73* |
| Unknown HIV status and/or previous TB treatment status | 0.96 (0.47-2.0) | *0.91* |

## 5.4 Discussion and conclusion

In Khayelitsha, the prevalence of routinely diagnosed RR-TB (including RMR- and MDR-TB), remained relatively stable from 2008 to 2017 inclusive, with no major temporal trend observed. Data from the study cohort (2013 to 2015 inclusive) showed that at the time of RR-TB diagnosis, there was no association between RMR-TB and HIV infection. However, RMR-TB was more likely to occur among HIV positive individuals who were HIV positive during previous first-line TB treatment, compared to both those who were HIV negative during previous TB treatment and those without previous TB treatment history. This suggests that there may be a higher risk of RIF R acquisition during first-line TB treatment among HIV positive individuals compared to those who are HIV negative.

A similar finding was found in a study conducted using data from 1998 to 2014, from the United States National TB Surveillance System by 49 states and the District of Columbia (excluding California due to gaps of HIV reporting to the CDC [Centers for disease control and prevention]) [262]. Data analysis from all *M.tb* culture positive cases suggested that individuals with HIV (at the time of RR-TB diagnosis), especially those with previous TB treatment, were more likely to have RMR-TB at the time of initial drug susceptibility testing (at the time of diagnosis). Furthermore, the percentage of RMR-TB among all culture positive TB cases (126 431) was 0.28% (359); and among these, the percentage of RMR-TB cases with HIV decreased yearly by 4% between 1998 and 2014. Nonetheless, the study found that all forms of RIF R were associated with HIV infection (compared to HIV negative individuals). Also, RIF R was associated with increased mortality between 1998 to 2014, controlling for HIV and other variables included in the study [262]. Also, another study conducted from 1993 to 2008 in California, found increased mortality of RMR-TB among individuals co-infected with HIV and TB when compared to drug sensitive TB [230].

Moreover, a systematic review and meta-analysis suggested that HIV infection was associated with a greater risk of RIF R acquisition [37]. Similarly, Munsiff *et al.* [238] observed a higher prevalence of

RMR-TB among HIV-TB co-infected cases compared to HIV negative cases by increased RIF R acquisition during TB treatment. However, this correlation is inconsistent across different geographical settings, and was not seen in this current research study from Khayelitsha.

To reiterate the findings from the systematic review within this book (Chapter 4), there are a number of possible factors that may contribute to RIF R acquisition in HIV positive individuals. The first possibility indicates that RR-TB infection among immunocompromised HIV positive patients has been associated with lower CD4 counts, which in turn is associated with significant gastrointestinal symptoms i.e. vomiting and diarrhoea; and changes in gut permeability in these patients [233, 238, 241]. Thus, this may lead to malabsorption of TB drugs, causing a greater risk of RIF R acquisition [48, 49]. Secondly, drug to drug interactions among HIV positive individuals receiving ART, may result in altering of pharmacokinetics of anti-TB drug medications [240, 251]. Hence, a few studies have shown that gastrointestinal symptoms, malabsorption, or drug-drug interactions with ART in combination with TB drug regimens, could lead to sub-therapeutic serum concentrations for one or more drugs [48-50, 240]. Lastly, extrapulmonary TB or disseminated TB disease may result in a higher bacterial load in immunocompromised, HIV-TB co-infected patients, leading to a greater chance of spontaneous mutations conferring RIF R being selected for during treatment. Another possibility is poor absorption of TB drugs as they are distributed at different concentrations to extrapulmonary compartments, resulting in the development of RR-TB [37, 240, 241].

While this study cohort from Khayelitsha showed an effect of HIV infection during previous first-line TB treatment, it is limited by the overall number of patients included, particularly in relation to ART during previous TB treatment. Another limitation within this study cohort is the lack of isoniazid mono-resistant TB (HMR-TB), that might have shown similarities to the acquisition of RMR-TB found in HIV positive individuals. Further research is needed to investigate this theory. There is also more evidence suggesting that the rifampicin dose recommended for both HIV positive and negative individuals may be too low and can be safely increased, when compared to the dosing of isoniazid [263-265]. Although the outcome of previous TB treatment was available for most (but not all) patients, the overall number of patients included was insufficient to differentiate between previous episode outcome and RMR-TB. In addition, data from randomized controlled trials (RCTs) are lacking in order to determine whether there is a RIF resistance amplification effect due to HIV. Thus, this study highlights the importance of conducting epidemiological studies, by accessing large datasets such as the PHDC as in this research study, for addressing questions to this effect and its impact on RIF R acquisition. Further research in this area is needed on a global scale to address these questions as RR-TB is an ongoing health concern worldwide. In general, cured and completed TB treatment outcomes are much lower in RR-TB patients than for rifampicin-susceptible TB (RS-TB) patients, resulting in poorer outcomes with higher mortality rates in these patients [2, 38]. With this said, in Khayelitsha, treatment outcomes remain relatively poor, mostly due to high loss to follow-up during treatment [192, 266]. Moreover, RR-TB is associated with higher costs to health systems globally, in addition to prolonged TB treatment and considerable drug toxicity in patients [230, 267-270].

Overall, the data presented suggest that HIV during previous first-line TB treatment may be associated with acquired rifampicin-resistance acquisition. Future prospective analysis will be required over a longer time period to further explore this in our study and in other studies. The data in this part of the study highlights the importance of preventing RR-TB by more effective treatment of TB among HIV positive individuals. Additionally, patient centred care could result in improved patient outcomes among both drug susceptible and drug resistant TB [192]. Also, prompt diagnosis of HIV-TB co-infection in patients, together with earlier ART initiation may prevent RIF R amplification.

# CHAPTER SIX

# 6. Mutations in *rpoB* and MICs among RR-TB strains (Results)

This chapter describes a study assessing the relationship between *rpoB* mutations determined by whole genome sequencing (WGS); and minimum inhibitory concentrations (MICs) determined by quantitative phenotypic drug susceptibility testing (q pDST); among rifampicin-resistant TB (RR-TB) strains in Khayelitsha. In this study, the phrase "RR-TB patients routinely diagnosed" refers to the initial, routine National Health Laboratory Service (NHLS) results. Rifampicin resistance (RIF R) was either diagnosed by GeneXpert MTB/RIF (Xpert) directly on specimens, or from a cultured isolate using a Genotype MTBDR*plus* line probe assay (LPA), and/or pDST with a mycobacterial growth indicator tube (MGIT). For this study, specimens from routinely diagnosed RR-TB patients were stored in a biobank, and when needed, isolates were re-cultured (in MGIT media) and tested at different time points by WGS and q pDST. Refer to Chapter 3 (section 3.8 and 3.9) for a full description of methods used in this chapter.

## 6.1 WGS-derived results: Overview

Between 2013 and 2015 inclusive, 670 RR-TB patients were routinely diagnosed with either Xpert and/or LPA. Figure 6.1 shows WGS-derived results.

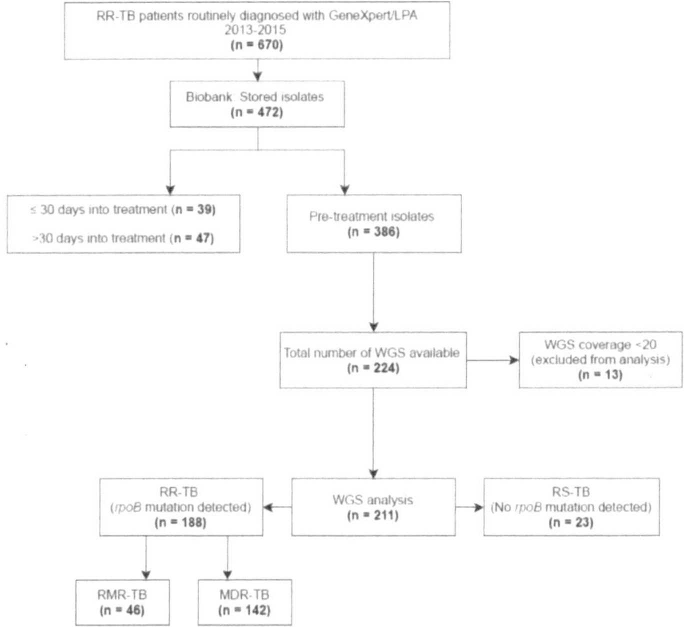


**Figure 6. 1** An overview of the total number of RR-TB patients routinely diagnosed with Xpert/LPA (n=670) during 2013-15 and the total number of WGS available for analysis (n=211), derived from stored pre-treatment isolates

Overall, 472/670 (70%) isolates were collected for research purposes and are currently stored in a biobank at Stellenbosch University (SU). The remaining 198/670 (30%) isolates were not stored; likely because of the following reasons. Firstly, some RR-TB patients only had one sputum sample available for Xpert testing and therefore no cultured isolate was available for storage. Secondly, some of the cultures were lost in the process due to cultures that were negative or contaminated. Lastly, several RR-TB patients without stored isolates did not start treatment, which reduced the possibility of later cultured isolates for storage.

Among the stored 472 RR-TB isolates, 386 were pre-treatment (i.e. the sputum sample was taken before second-line treatment was initiated). The remainder were not pre-treatment isolates, as 39 were sputum samples that were taken ≤30 days into treatment, and 47 were sputum samples taken >30 days into treatment. However, of the 386 pre-treatment isolates, only 224 (58%) WGS results were available for further analysis during the time of the study. Refer to Table 6.1 for reasons as to why sequencing results were not available and/or in progress during the analysis phase at the time of this study.

**Table 6. 1** Main reasons for the remainder of stored pre-treatment isolates (162/386; 42%); from RR-TB patients routinely diagnosed during 2013-15 in Khayelitsha; that were not available for further analysis in this study

| **Reasons** | **Total (n = 162)** |
|---|---|
| Negative (upon re-culture) | 12 |
| Contaminated (upon re-culture) | 11 |
| Sample missing (from stored isolates) | 1 |
| *WGS pending | 138 |
| ***Total*** | **162** |

*Stored isolates were either re-cultured (n=45) or in the process of DNA extraction (n=38) or DNA was sent to Switzerland to perform WGS (n=55)

WGS coverage relative to the reference genome of at least 20x was obtained in more than 94% of WGS samples (211/224) [120, 210]. Refer to Chapter 3 (Methodology) for commonly used parameters used for the WGS analysis pipeline. Thus, 211 routinely diagnosed stored RR-TB strains had WGS data available for further analysis (Figure 6.2).

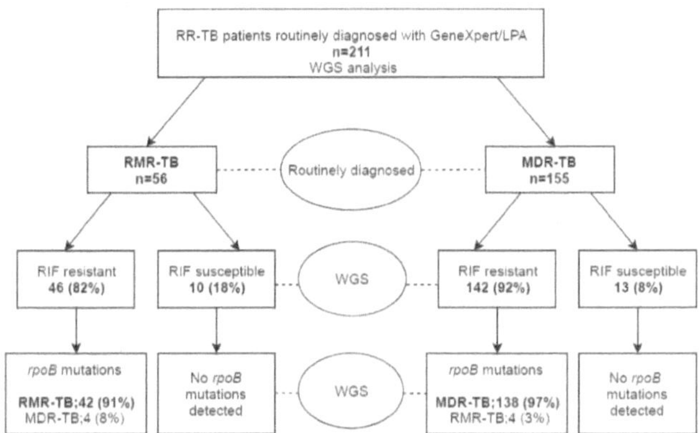


**Figure 6. 2** An illustration of WGS results of 211 RR-TB stored isolates, derived from patients who were routinely diagnosed with Xpert/LPA during 2013-15

Among the 211 routinely diagnosed stored RR-TB strains, 56 (27%) were rifampicin mono-resistant TB (RMR-TB) and 155 (73%) were multi-drug resistant TB (MDR-TB) according to routine diagnostic results (Figure 6.2). Among the routine RMR-TB strains, considerable discordance with WGS data was found; 10/56 (18%) were RIF susceptible TB (RS-TB) with no RIF R conferring *rpoB* mutations detected. This was significantly higher than the discordance found among routinely diagnosed MDR-TB that were RS-TB according to WGS (p=0.03).

Among the routine RMR-TB strains with RIF R conferring *rpoB* mutations detected with WGS, 4 (8%) were resistant to both RIF and INH, and were therefore MDR-TB; while the remainder were INH susceptible (91%) and therefore had confirmed RMR-TB (Figure 6.2).

WGS-derived results showed RR-TB with RIF R conferring *rpoB* mutations [188/211 (89%)], of which 46 were RMR-TB (24%) and 142 were MDR-TB (76%), respectively. Discordance (11%; 23/211) was found among the remaining WGS-derived results showing RS-TB; even though these were TB isolates from routinely diagnosed RR-TB patients. The results of all 23 WGS-derived RS-TB strains are illustrated below (section 6.2).

## 6.2 Discordance (RS-TB with WGS)

Among the 23 routinely diagnosed RR-TB patients with RS-TB on WGS (with no RIF R conferring *rpoB* mutations), 10 (43%) were routinely diagnosed with RMR-TB and 13 (57%) with MDR-TB (Figure 6.3). Among the 10 routinely diagnosed RMR-TB strains, considerable discordance was found in 8/10 (80%) strains showing RS-TB according to both WGS and q pDST results (Figure 6.3). Among the 13 routinely diagnosed MDR-TB strains, 6/13 (46%) were phenotypically susceptible, while 4/13 (31%) were phenotypically resistant (Figure 6.3). The remaining 3/13 (23%) isolates failed to grow (no growth) in the MGIT (Figure 6.3).

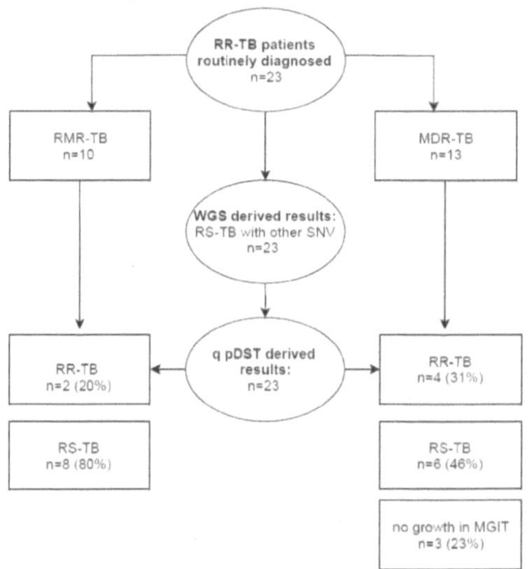


**Figure 6. 3** A diagrammatic representation of results produced from WGS-derived RS-TB as well as q pDST among 23 routinely diagnosed RR-TB patients with discordant results.

Table 6.2 provides detailed results for the 23 routinely diagnosed RR-TB patients; including WGS and q pDST; that were re-cultured (in MGITs) from stored isolates. All 23 RR-TB patients presented with culture positive *M.tb*, and 10 patients had smear-negative results (Table 6.2). All 23 RR-TB patients were routinely diagnosed with the LPA, while 15 patients were routinely diagnosed with both Xpert and LPA (Table 6.2). WGS results showed that 74% (17/23) of RS-TB strains had *rpoB* small single nucleotide variants (SNV) that are not known to confer RIF R (these isolates were not classified as RR-TB by WGS - TB profiler) (Table 6.2). Of these, the majority (13/17; 76%) were synonymous silent mutations (Table 6.2).

Potential reasons for discordance were based on differences found between the initial routine diagnostic results, q pDST and WGS results described in Table 6.2. In this study, potential reasons for discordance found among the 23 routinely diagnosed RR-TB patients (Table 6.2) may have resulted from either mixed infection (43%), false-positive RIF R (18%), or both (39%) (Figure 6.4). Below is the approach and terminology used in this part of the study to categorise between discordances found:

- **False-positive RIF R:** Patients that were routinely diagnosed with RR-TB by Xpert and/or LPA. Subsequent WGS testing from patient stored isolates showed RS-TB (no RIF resistance conferring mutations found) with synonymous silent mutations detected, indicating the possibility of false-positive RIF R. Further testing with the MGIT also showed RS-TB, further indicating the possibility of false-positive RIF R.

- **Mixed infection:** Patients that were routinely diagnosed with RR-TB by Xpert and/or LPA. Subsequent WGS testing from patient stored isolates showed RS-TB, mostly without SNV (6/10) or *rpoB* SNV mutation frequencies ≤41% (3/10). Further testing with the MGIT mostly showed RS-TB (7/10). A mixture of RR-TB and RS-TB isolates may have resulted in the discordant DST results seen.
- **Mixed infection and/or false positive RIF R:** Patients that were routinely diagnosed with RR-TB by Xpert and/or LPA. Subsequent WGS testing from patient stored isolates resulted in RS-TB with either synonymous silent mutations indicating the possibility of false-positive RIF R (7/9) or RS-TB strains with different lineages/sublineages, suggestive of a mixed infection (2/9). Further testing with the MGIT showed RR-TB or RS-TB indicating the possibility of mixed infections.

**Table 6. 2** A detailed layout of discordant results found among 23 routinely diagnosed RR-TB patient results (from NHLS), compared with q pDST and WGS-derived results (both from re-cultured stored isolates), performed at different time intervals throughout the study.

| | Routine diagnostic results (RR-TB); (all culture positive) | | | q pDST-derived results (MGIT) | | WGS-derived results (RS-TB) | | | | Potential reasons for discordance |
|---|---|---|---|---|---|---|---|---|---|---|
| **Study ID** | **Smear result** | **GeneXpert (RIF R/S) (time1=initial diagnosis)** | **LPA results (time1=initial diagnosis)** | **RIF MIC (µg/ml)** | **INH MIC (µg/ml)** | **WGS-derived: No RIF R conferring mutations detected by TB profiler** | **Other *rpoB* SNV manually detected by TB profiler and Artemis sequence viewer (mutation frequency)** | **Type of SNV *rpoB* mutation** | **WGS strain lineage (TB profiler)** | **Discordance based on routine, MGIT and WGS-derived results** |
| ***RMR-TB routinely diagnosed patients that tested RS-TB with both WGS & q pDST stored isolates (n=8)*** | | | | | | | | | | |
| TB999 | Neg | R (time1) | ➢ RIF R; INH S (time1 plus 6days) | 0.5 (RIF S) | 0.1 (INH S) | RS-TB (RIF S; INH S) | *rpoB* A1075A "c.3225T>C" (100%) | synonymous silent mutation | lineage2.2.1.1; East Asian (Beijing) | **False-positive RIF R** (Xpert; LPA) |
| TB998 | Neg | ND | ➢ RIF R; INH S (time1) | 0.5 (RIF S) | 0.1 (INH S) | RS-TB (RIF S; INH S) | *rpoB* A1075A "c.3225T>C" (100%) | synonymous silent mutation | lineage4.[illegible]; Euro-American (mainly T) | **False-positive RIF R** (LPA) |
| TB997 | ND | ND | ➢ RIF R; INH S (time1) | 0.5 (RIF S) | 0.1 (INH S) | RS-TB (RIF S; INH S) | *rpoB* A1075A "c.3225T>C" (100%) | synonymous silent mutation | lineage4.[illegible]; Euro-American (mainly T) | **False-positive RIF R** (LPA) |
| TB996 | ND | S (time1) | ➢ RIF R; INH S (time1)<br>➢ Susceptible (time1 plus 6days) | 0.5 (RIF S) | 0.1 (INH S) | RS-TB (RIF S; INH S) | None | NA | lineage4.3.2.1; Euro-American (LAM) | **Mixed infection** (RR-TB; RS-TB) |
| TB995 | Neg | R (time1) | ➢ RIF R; INH S (time1) | 0.5 (RIF S) | 0.1 (INH S) | RS-TB (RIF S; INH S) | None | NA | lineage4.3.2.1; Euro-American (LAM) | **Mixed infection** (RR-TB; RS-TB) |
| TB994 | 3+ | ND | ➢ RIF R; INH S (time1); | 0.5 (RIF S) | 0.1 (INH S) | RS-TB (RIF S; INH S) | *rpoB* T1018A "p.Thr1018Ala" ***(25%)** | nonsynonymous missense mutation | lineage2.2.[illegible]1; | **Mixed infection** (RR-TB; RS-TB) |

| | | | | | | | | | | |
|---|---|---|---|---|---|---|---|---|---|---|
| | | | ➢ Susceptible (time1 plus 10days) | | | | | | East Asian (Beijing) | |
| TB993 | 3+ | R (time1) | ➢ RIF R; INH S (time1);<br>➢ RIF R; INH S (time1 plus 11days) | 0.5 (RIF S) | 0.1 (INH S) | RS-TB (RIF S; INH S) | *rpoB* T1018A "p.Thr1018Ala" ***(41%)** | nonsynonymous missense mutation | lineage2.2.1; East Asian (Beijing) | **Mixed infection** (RR-TB; RS-TB) |
| TB992 | Neg | ND | ➢ RIF R; INH S (time1) | 0.5 (RIF S) | 0.1 (INH S) | RS-TB (RIF S; INH S) | *rpoB* 130T "c.390C>T" (85%) | synonymous silent mutation | lineage4.1.1.1; Euro-American (X-type) and lineage4.3.3; Euro-American (LAM) | **Mixed infection** (different sub-lineages) **and/or false-positive RIF R** (LPA) |
| ***RMR-TB routinely diagnosed patients that tested RR-TB with q pDST but RS-TB with WGS stored isolates (n=2)*** | | | | | | | | | | |
| TB991 | 1+ | ND | ➢ RIF R; INH S (time1) | 2 (RIF R) | 0.1 (INH S) | RS-TB (RIF S; INH S) | None | NA | lineage4.1.1 Euro-American (X-type) | **Mixed infection** (RR-TB; RS-TB) |
| TB990 | 1+ | R (time1) | ➢ RIF R; INH S (time1) | 2 (RIF R) | 0.1 (INH S) | HMR-TB *katG_p.Trp191Arg (100%);* (RIF S; INH R) | *rpoB* A1075A "c.3225T>C" (100%) | synonymous silent mutation | lineage2.2.1.1 East Asian (Beijing) | **Mixed infection** (RR-TB; RS-TB) **and/or false-positive RIF R** (Xpert; LPA) |
| ***MDR-TB routinely diagnosed patients that tested RS-TB with both WGS & q pDST stored isolates (n=6)*** | | | | | | | | | | |
| TB989 | Neg | ND | ➢ RIF R; INH R (time1) | 0.5 (RIF S) | 0.1 (INH S) | RS-TB (RIF S; INH S) | *rpoB* A1075A "c.3225T>C" (100%) | synonymous silent mutation | lineage2.2.1 East Asian (Beijing) | **False-positive RIF R** (LPA) |
| TB988 | Neg | R (time1) | ➢ RIF R; INH R (time1); | 0.5 (RIF S) | 0.1 (INH S) | RS-TB (RIF S; INH S) | None | NA | lineage4.1.1.3 Euro-American (X-type) | **Mixed infection** (RR-TB; RS-TB) |

| | | | ➢ RIF R; INH R (time1 plus 8days) | | | | | | | |
|---|---|---|---|---|---|---|---|---|---|---|
| TB987 | Neg | R (time1) | ➢ RIF R; INH R (time1);<br>➢ RIF R; INH R (time1 plus 6days);<br>➢ RIF R; INH R (time1 plus 13 days) | 1 (RIF S) | 0.1 (INH S) | RS-TB<br>(RIF S; INH S) | None | NA | lineage4.3.2.1<br>Euro-American<br>(LAM) | **Mixed infection**<br>(RR-TB; RS-TB) |
| TB986 | ND | ND | ➢ RIF R; INH R (time1) | 1 (RIF S) | 0.1 (INH S) | HMR-TB<br>*fabG1_c.-15C>T (100%);*<br>(RIF S; INH R) | *rpoB* A1075A "c.3225T>C" (100%) | synonymous silent mutation | lineage2.2.1<br>East Asian<br>(Beijing) | **Mixed infection**<br>(RR-TB; HMR-TB)<br>**and/or false-positive RIF R** (LPA) |
| TB985 | 3+ | R (time1) | ➢ RIF R; INH R (time1) | 0.5 (RIF S) | >1 (INH R) | HMR-TB<br>*inhA_p.Gly40Trp*<br>***(13%)**<br>(RIF S; INH R) | *rpoB* T1018A "p.Thr1018Ala" ***(21%)** | nonsynonymous missense mutation | lineage4.3.2.1<br>Euro-American<br>(LAM) | **Mixed infection**<br>(RR-TB; HMR-TB) |
| TB984 | Neg | R (time1) | ➢ RIF R; INH R (time1) | 1 (RIF S) | 1 (INH R) | RS-TB<br>(RIF S; INH S) | *rpoB* A1075A "c.3225T>C" ***(56%)** | synonymous silent mutation | lineage4.3.2.1;<br>Euro-American<br>(LAM) and<br>lineage2.2;<br>East Asian<br>(Beijing) | **Mixed infection**<br>(RR-TB; HMR-TB);<br>(different lineages)<br>**and/or false-positive RIF R**<br>(Xpert; LPA) |
| ***MDR-TB routinely diagnosed patients that tested RR-TB with q pDST but RS-TB with WGS stored isolates (n=4)*** | | | | | | | | | | |
| TB983 | 1+ | R (time1) | ➢ RIF R; INH R (time1) | 2 (RIF R) | 1 (INH R) | HMR-TB<br>*katG_c.1046_1046del*<br>***(12%)** | *rpoB* V262A " p.Val262Ala"(100%) | nonsynonymous missense mutation | lineage4.4.1.1<br>Euro-American<br>(S-type) | **Mixed infection**<br>(RR-TB; HMR-TB) |

| | | | | | | | | | | |
|---|---|---|---|---|---|---|---|---|---|---|
| | | | ➢ RIF R; INH R (time1 plus 7days) | | | (RIF S; INH R) | | | | |
| TB982 | Neg | ND | ➢ RIF R; INH R (time1)<br>➢ RIF R; INH R (time1 plus 6days) | 10 (RIF R) | >1 (INH R) | RS-TB (RIF S; INH S) | *rpoB* A1075A "c.3225T>C" (100%) | synonymous silent mutation | lineage4.6.1.1 Euro-American (T2) | **Mixed infection** (RR-TB; RS-TB) **and/or false-positive RIF R** (LPA) |
| TB981 | Neg | R (time1) | ➢ Susceptible (time1)<br>➢ RIF R; INH R (time1 plus 11 days)<br>➢ Susceptible (time1 plus 34days) | 10 (RIF R) | 0.1 (INH S) | RS-TB (RIF S; INH S) | *rpoB* A1075A "c.3225T>C" (99%) | synonymous silent mutation | lineage2.2.1.1 East Asian (Beijing) | **Mixed infection** (RR-TB; RS-TB) **and/or false-positive RIF R** (Xpert; LPA) |
| TB980 | 1+ | R (time1) | ➢ RIF R; INH R (time1)<br>➢ RIF R; INH R (time1 plus 4days) | 10 (RIF R) | >1 (INH R) | RS-TB (RIF S; INH S) | *rpoB* A1075A "c.3225T>C" (100%) | synonymous silent mutation | lineage2.2.1.1 East Asian (Beijing) | **Mixed infection** (RR-TB; RS-TB) **and/or false-positive RIF R** (Xpert; LPA) |
| ***MDR-TB routinely diagnosed patients that tested RS-TB with WGS stored isolates; whereas q pDST MGITs failed to grow (n=3)*** | | | | | | | | | | |
| TB979 | 3+ | R (time1) | ➢ RIF R; INH R (time1<br>➢ RIF R; INH R (time1 plus 24days) | No growth | No growth | HMR-TB *fabG1_c.-15C>T (100%)* (RIF S; INH R) | None | NA | lineage2.2.1 East Asian (Beijing) | **Mixed infection** (RR-TB; HMR-TB) |
| TB978 | 3+ | R (time1)<br>R (time1 plus 2days) | ➢ RIF R; INH R (time1) | No growth | No growth | HMR-TB *fabG1_c.-15C>T,* | *rpoB* A1075A "c.3225T>C" (100%) | synonymous silent mutation | lineage2.2.1.1 East Asian (Beijing) | **Mixed infection** (RR-TB; HMR-TB) **and/or false-** |

| | | | | | | | | | | |
|---|---|---|---|---|---|---|---|---|---|---|
| | | | ➤ RIF S; INH R [HMR-TB] (time1 plus 2days) | | | *inhA_p.Ser94Ala* *(100%)* (RIF S; INH R) | | | | **positive RIF R** (Xpert; LPA) |
| TB977 | 3+ | R (time1) | ➤ RIF R; INH R (time1)<br>➤ RIF S; INH R [HMR-TB] (time1 plus 7days) | No growth | No growth | RS-TB (RIF S; INH S) | *rpoB* 876G "c.2628T>G" (96%) | synonymous silent mutation | lineage3.1.1 East-African-Indian (CAS) | **Mixed infection** (RR-TB; HMR-TB) **and/or false-positive RIF R** (Xpert; LPA) |

**Note:** * Mutation frequencies that are low; **Abbreviations:** LPA (Line probe assay); R (resistant); RIF R (Rifampicin resistance); S (Susceptible); RIF S (Rifampicin susceptible); RS-TB (Rifampicin susceptible TB); Neg – (Negative); ND (Not done); NA (Not applicable); HMR-TB (Isoniazid mono-resistant TB); SNV (small single nucleotide variants); **Definitions:** RS-TB = No rifampicin resistance conferring mutations detected with WGS; time1 = Timepoint of the initial routine diagnostic results (from NLHS) (i.e. the first time DR-TB was routinely identified on either the GeneXpert and/or LPA)

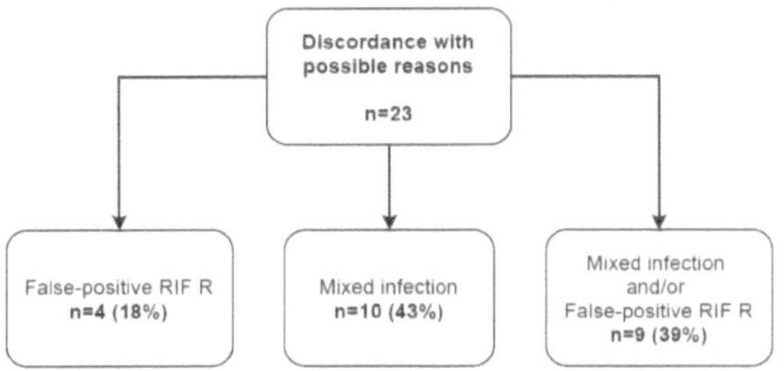


**Figure 6. 4** A summary of the possible reasons for discordance found among 23 routinely diagnosed RR-TB patient results (from NHLS), compared with q pDST and WGS-derived results (both from re-cultured stored isolates), performed at different time intervals throughout the study

**Note:** Refer to Table 6.2 for a detailed layout

## 6.3 Distribution of *rpoB* mutations (RR-TB with WGS)

The *Escherichia coli (E. coli)* gene nomenclature for naming *rpoB* mutations was used throughout this study [20]. Refer to Table 6.4 for reference to the *M.tb* complex numbering system in this study [23]. The tables below illustrate the differences between RMR- and MDR-TB strains and their associated confidence assessment for the 188 RR-TB strains that showed RIF R conferring *rpoB* mutations on WGS. The number of minimal confidence *rpoB* mutations were significantly higher among RMR-TB than for MDR-TB; when compared to high/moderate confidence *rpoB* mutations (p=0.002) (Table 6.3).

**Table 6. 3** WGS-based *rpoB* mutations with confidence levels conferring RIF R among RMR- and MDR-TB strains (n=188)

| ***rpoB* mutation confidence level *** | **RMR-TB (WGS) n = 46 (%)** | **MDR-TB (WGS) n = 142 (%)** | **Total n = 188 (%)** |
|---|---|---|---|
| High/Moderate | 38 (83%) | 134 (94%) | 172 (91%) |
| Minimal | 8 (17%) | 5 (4%) | 13 (7%) |
| Not classified | 0 (0%) | 3 (2%) | 3 (2%) |
| ***Total*** | ***46*** | ***142*** | ***188*** |

* Confidence levels were reported by Miotto *et al.* [147]; however, if not reported these were referred to as 'not classified' in this study.

**Table 6. 4** WGS-based RIF R conferring *rpoB* mutations in the order of high to not classified confidence levels found among RMR- and MDR-TB strains (n=188)

| *rpoB* mutation (WGS) | RMR-TB (WGS) n = 46 | MDR-TB (WGS) n = 142 | *rpoB* mutation confidence level * |
|---|---|---|---|
| S531L (S450L) | 13 (28%) | 100 (70%) | High |
| S531F (S450F) | 0 | 1 | High |
| H526Y (H445Y) | 10 (22%) | 7 (5%) | High |
| H526D (H445D) | 3 | 5 | High |
| H526L (H445L) | 1 | 2 | High |
| D516V (D435V) | 0 | 11 | High |
| D516F (D435F) | 4 | 0 | High |
| D516G (D435G) | 1 | 0 | High |
| Q513K (Q432K) | 0 | 2 | High |
| L533P (L452P) | 2 | 4 | Moderate |
| S522L (S441L) | 2 | 0 | Moderate |
| D516Y (D435Y) | 2 | 2 | Moderate |
| I572F (I491F) | 0 | 1 | Minimal |
| H526N (H445N) | 0 | 2 | Minimal |
| L511P (L430P) | 8 (17%) | 2 (1.4%) | Minimal |
| V146F (V170F) | 0 | 1 | Not classified |
| T481A (T400A) | 0 | 2 | Not classified |

**Note:** The first *rpoB* mutation (e.g S531L) is according to *E. coli* nomenclature, whereas the second *rpoB* mutation (e.g S450L) is according to the *M.tb* complex numbering system. *Confidence levels were reported by Miotto *et al.* [147] however, if not reported these were referred to as 'not classified' in this study.

Among the 46 RMR-TB strains (by WGS), the most common *rpoB* mutations were S531L (n = 13; 28%), followed by both H526Y (n = 10; 22%) and L511P (n = 8; 17%) (Table 6.4). L511P was reported as the only minimal confidence *rpoB* mutation conferring RIF resistance among all RMR-TB strains. Overall, a total of 38/46 (83%) RMR-TB strains had *rpoB* mutations with high/moderate confidence in conferring rifampicin-resistance (Table 6.3).

Among the 142 MDR-TB strains (by WGS), *rpoB* S531L (high confidence) was found in 70% (100/143) of MDR-TB strains. In contrast to RMR-TB, the L511P mutation was present in only 1.4% (2/143) MDR-TB strains (p<0.01, compared to RMR-TB) (Table 6.4). Interestingly, there were three MDR-TB strains with *rpoB* mutations conferring rifampicin resistance outside the rifampicin resistance determining region (RRDR) of the *rpoB* gene (i.e. I572F, T481A, V146F); these mutations were not seen among WGS-derived RMR-TB strains.

### 6.3.1 Relationship between *rpoB* mutations (WGS) and MICs (q pDST)

q pDST was performed for all minimal, moderate and confidence level *rpoB* mutations that were 'not classified' by Miotto *et al.* [147], among the 188 WGS-derived RR-TB strains. Additionally, q pDST was performed on strains found to be RS-TB with WGS but were isolated from patients routinely diagnosed with RR-TB.

In total, 51 strains were phenotypically tested with the MGIT. These included 28 RR-TB and 23 RS-TB strains based on WGS. RR-TB tested by q pDST included 13 (46%) minimal, 12 (43%) moderate and 3 (11%) 'not classified' confidence levels for RIF R, respectively [147].

- ***Strains with minimal confidence level rpoB mutations (WGS-based)***

Interestingly, all 10 *rpoB* L511P strains (8 RMR-TB; 2 MDR-TB), tested phenotypically susceptible to rifampicin in the MGIT at the critical concentration or lower (RIF MIC = ≤ 1 µg/ml) (Table 6.5). Among MDR-TB, two H526N strains (minimal confidence) tested phenotypically resistant (Table 6.6). However, the remaining one MDR-TB strain with I572F tested phenotypically susceptible to rifampicin in the MGIT (Table 6.6).

**Table 6. 5** q pDST MIC levels for rifampicin and isoniazid among isolates with minimal confidence *rpoB* L511P mutations (n=10)

| ***rpoB* mutation(s)** | **WGS DR-TB profile** | **Rifampicin MIC** | **Isoniazid MIC** | **q pDST profile** | **Number of strains** |
|---|---|---|---|---|---|
| L511P | RMR | **0.25 µg/ml *** | **0.1 µg/ml *** | RIF-S; INH-S | 2 |
| L511P | RMR | **0.125 µg/ml *** | **0.1 µg/ml *** | RIF-S; INH-S | 4 |
| L511P | RMR | **0.5 µg/ml *** | **0.1 µg/ml *** | RIF-S; INH-S | 1 |
| L511P | RMR | **1 µg/ml *** | **0.1 µg/ml *** | RIF-S; INH-S | 1 |
| L511P | MDR | **1 µg/ml *** | 1 µg/ml | RIF-S; INH-R | 2 |

**Note:** * Susceptible

**Table 6. 6** q pDST MIC levels for rifampicin and isoniazid among the remaining isolates with minimal confidence *rpoB* mutations (n=3)

| ***rpoB* mutation(s)** | **WGS DR-TB profile** | **Rifampicin MIC** | **Isoniazid MIC** | **q pDST profile** | **Number of strains** |
|---|---|---|---|---|---|
| H526N | MDR | 20 µg/ml | 1 µg/ml | RIF-R; INH-R | 2 |
| I572F | MDR | **1 µg/ml *** | 1 µg/ml | RIF-S; INH-R | 1 |

**Note:** * Susceptible

- ***Strains with moderate confidence level rpoB mutations (WGS-based)***

The 2 RMR-TB strains with *rpoB* mutations D516Y and L533P, tested phenotypically susceptible to rifampicin in the MGIT (Table 6.7). However, all MDR-TB strains with D516Y (n=2) and L533P (n=4) tested phenotypically resistant to both rifampicin and isoniazid. The 2 RMR-TB strains with *rpoB* S522L were phenotypically resistant to rifampicin (Table 6.7).

**Table 6. 7** q pDST MIC levels for rifampicin and isoniazid among moderate confidence *rpoB* mutations (n=12)

| ***rpoB* mutation(s)** | **WGS DR-TB profile** | **Rifampicin MIC** | **Isoniazid MIC** | **q pDST profile** | **Number of strains** |
|---|---|---|---|---|---|
| S522L | RMR | 10 µg/ml | **0.1 µg/ml *** | RIF-R; INH-S | 2 |
| D516Y | RMR | **1 µg/ml *** | 1 µg/ml | RIF-S; INH-R | 2 |
| D516Y | MDR | 2 µg/ml | 1 µg/ml | RIF-R; INH-R | 2 |
| L533P | RMR | **0.5 µg/ml *** | **0.1 µg/ml *** | RIF-S; INH-S | 2 |
| L533P | MDR | 2 µg/ml | 1 µg/ml | RIF-R; INH-R | 3 |
| L533P | MDR | 10 µg/ml | 1 µg/ml | RIF-R; INH-R | 1 |

**Note:** * Susceptible

- ***Strains with confidence level rpoB mutations not classified (WGS-based)***

All MDR-TB strains with V146F and T481A *rpoB* mutations were phenotypically resistant to rifampicin with MIC ranges between 10-20 µg/ml (Table 6.8).

**Table 6. 8** q pDST MIC levels for rifampicin and isoniazid among confidence level *rpoB* mutations that were not classified (n=3)

| ***rpoB* mutation(s)** | **WGS DR-TB profile** | **Rifampicin MIC** | **Isoniazid MIC** | **q pDST profile** | **Number of strains** |
|---|---|---|---|---|---|
| V146F | MDR | 20 µg/ml | 1 µg/ml | RIF-R; INH-R | 1 |
| T481A | MDR | 10 µg/ml | 1 µg/ml | RIF-R; INH-R | 1 |
| T481A | MDR | 20 µg/ml | 1 µg/ml | RIF-R; INH-R | 1 |

## 6.4 DR-TB profiles (RR-TB with WGS)

Table 6.9 shows a summary of the DR-TB profiles obtained for all 188 RR-TB strains derived by WGS. The table highlights that all 46 WGS-derived RMR-TB strains were resistant to rifampicin only; with no other *M.tb* drug resistance. Among WGS-derived MDR-TB strains, 38 different DR-TB profiles were found; these are described separately by fluoroquinolone susceptibility (Table 6.9).

**Table 6. 9** Frequency of the different WGS-derived (TB profiler) DR-TB profiles among 188 routinely diagnosed RR-TB patients in Khayelitsha across 2013-15

| **Resistance profile (WGS-based)** | **Number of strains** |
|---|---|
| Rifampicin-susceptible TB (no *rpoB* mutations) | 23 |
| Rifampicin-resistant TB (*rpoB* mutations) | 188 |
| **RMR-TB (n = 46, 24%)** | |
| R | 46 |
| **MDR-TB (FLQ susceptible) (n = 123, 65%)** | |
| $H_{high}$R | 7 |
| $H_{high}$RESZ | 4 |
| $H_{high}$RE | 9 |
| $H_{high}$REZ | 2 |
| $H_{high}$RS | 10 |
| $H_{high}$RS, ETO | 2 |
| $H_{high}$RES | 8 |
| $H_{high}$RES AMI | 1 |
| $H_{high}$RZS | 2 |
| $H_{high}$RZS, ETO | 11 |
| $H_{high}$RZS, ETO, AMI | 4 |
| $H_{high}$RZ ETO | 1 |
| $H_{high}$R, ETO | 16 |
| $H_{high}$RE, ETO | 7 |
| $H_{high}$RES, ETO | 4 |
| $H_{high}$RES, ETO, AMI | 4 |
| $H_{high}$RES, ETO, AMI, CAP, KAN | 3 |
| $H_{high}$RESZ, ETO, AMI | 2 |
| $H_{high}$RESZ, ETO, AMI, CAP, KAN | 2 |
| $H_{high}$RZS, PAS | 1 |
| $H_{low}$R, ETO | 2 |
| $H_{low}$RE, ETO | 8 |
| $H_{low}$RESZ, ETO | 2 |
| $H_{low}$RESZ, ETO, AMI | 4 |
| $H_{low}$RESZ, ETO, AMI, KAN | 1 |
| $H_{low}$REZ, ETO | 6 |
| **MDR-TB (FLQ resistance n = 19, 10%)** | |
| $H_{low}$RE, ETO, FLQ | 1 |
| $H_{low}$REZ, ETO, FLQ | 1 |
| $H_{high}$RE ETO, FLQ | 1 |
| $H_{high}$RES, ETO FLQ, AMI | 1 |
| $H_{high}$RES, FLQ, AMI | 1 |
| $H_{high}$RES, ETO, FLQ, AMI, CAP, KAN | 1 |
| $H_{high}$RES, ETO, FLQ, PAS AMI, CAP, KAN | 1 |
| $H_{high}$RESZ, FLQ | 1 |
| $H_{high}$RESZ, ETO, FLQ, AMI | 2 |
| $H_{high}$RESZ, ETO, FLQ, AMI, CAP, KAN | 4 |

| $H_{high}$RESZ, FLQ, AMI, CAP, KAN | 2 |
|---|---|
| $H_{high}$RZS, ETO, FLQ | 3 |

**Abbreviations:** RS-TB = Rifampicin susceptible TB; RR-TB = Rifampicin-resistant TB; R = Rifampicin; $H_{high}$ = Isoniazid high level resistance (*katG* mutations); $H_{low}$ = Isoniazid low-level resistance (*inhA* mutations only); E = Ethambutol; S = Streptomycin; ETO = Ethionamide; Z = Pyrazinamide; FLQ = Fluoroquinolone; AMI = Amikacin; CAP = Capreomycin; KAN = Kanamycin

## CHAPTER SEVEN

# 7. Mutations in *rpoB* and MICs among RR-TB strains (Discussion)

## 7.1 Discussion

This part of the study provided an overview of *rpoB* mutations determined by whole genome sequencing (WGS); and minimum inhibitory concentrations (MICs) determined by quantitative phenotypic drug susceptibility testing (q pDST); among rifampicin-resistant TB (RR-TB) strains in Khayelitsha during 2013 to 2015. One of the key findings included a high proportion (11%) of strains with discordance found among rifampicin resistance (RIF R) routinely diagnosed RR-TB patients. WGS results (TB profiler) showed that the DR-TB profile for *rpoB* mutations were distinctly different between rifampicin mono-resistant TB (RMR-TB) and multi-drug resistant TB (MDR-TB) strains. Furthermore, the proportion of high/moderate versus minimal confidence levels for *rpoB* mutations was significantly higher among MDR-TB than for RMR-TB. Interestingly though, among RMR-TB strains, there was a significant difference in *rpoB* L511P; described as a disputed mutation, conferring minimal confidence for RIF R or low-level RIF R; 17% and 1.4% among RMR- and MDR-TB, respectively. In addition, all *rpoB* L511P mutations (including RMR- and MDR-TB) tested phenotypically susceptible to rifampicin (RS-TB) with the mycobacteria growth indicator tube (MGIT) q pDST; causing discrepancies between WGS and q pDST results. Lastly, all RMR-TB strains; including those with the L511P mutations; had no other mutations conferring resistance to any of the other TB drugs.

As initially stated, this part of the study found a relatively high number of strains (11%) with discordance in RIF R among routinely diagnosed RR-TB patients of which 43% were RMR-TB and 57% were MDR-TB. Subsequent WGS testing from these patients on re-cultured stored isolates, indicated RS-TB with no RIF R conferring mutations. Notably, WGS and qDST were often performed on different sub-cultures taken from stored stock. This may have selected for defined sub-populations of RR-TB and RS-TB in this study. Possible causes for discordance from these study findings were deemed as either mixed infections (43%), false-positive RIF R (18%) or both (39%). Heteroresistance may occur during the early stages of drug-resistant TB (DR-TB) development in patients, with co-existing subpopulations of RR-TB and RS-TB, or heteroresistance could be due to mixed infections, i.e. infection with more than one *Mycobacterium tuberculosis (M.tb)* strain [24, 59, 271-274]. Among the discordant results found in this study, only two WGS-derived RS-TB strains had a different lineage/sublineage, suggestive of potential mixed infections of strains. Also, among discordant mixed infections in this study, a small proportion of *rpoB* single nucleotide variants (SNV) had mutation frequencies ≤41%; suggestive of potential mixed populations of strains. In the past, it was reported that pDST could determine at least 1% or more of the bacterial population in clinical specimens that were DR-TB [98, 99]. Observations by Folkvardsen *et al.* [274] were that pDST was more sensitive and had better detection rates in identifying heteroresistance compared to molecular methods. Moreover, Zhang *et al.* [275] showed that the broth dilution method (not used in this study - Chapter six) was significantly more sensitive in detecting heteroresistance in RIF, in subpopulations with low growth rates compared to the liquid MGIT-DST method (used in this study - Chapter six). Moreover, previous studies have shown that mixed infections can result in discordance between pDST and mutation analysis results [271, 276, 277]. In other studies, phenotypically RR-TB isolates with no mutations [RS-TB] found by polymerase chain reaction (PCR) of the *rpoB* gene and sequencing, were reported in 5% [278] and 3.8% [277] of strains; with the latter study reporting a significant association with mixed infections [277]. Authors suggest that this could have been due to mutations of RR-TB isolates with mixed infections not detected by DNA sequencing, as they were performed on cultured isolates, and could therefore possibly contain mixed populations of strains, or even contaminating DNA [271]. Notably, a single sputum sample is not a complete representation of the overall diversity of a given *M.tb* strain. Thus, culturing an isolate could furthermore reduce the diversity of an *M.tb* strain [279, 280]. However, this could be resolved by performing deep sequencing or WGS to a series of isolates collected from the same patient, over different time points to determine the acquisition of mutations [281, 282].

Our understanding to date is that synonymous silent mutations in the *rpoB* gene, do not cause amino acid changes, have no phenotypic effect, and are not known to confer RIF R. Although some evidence does suggest the possibility of undiscovered complex effects on function related differences to synonymous silent mutations, this possibility needs further investigation to determine if there is an association with RIF R [283, 284]. However, among RR-TB isolates these silent mutations are detected as an absence of wild type probe; hence interpreted as RIF R or RR-TB on the GeneXpert MTB/RIF (Xpert) / GenoType MTBDR*plus* line probe assay (LPA), as described by various studies [273, 285-288]. Hence, these silent mutations do cause discordance between genotypic and phenotypic diagnostic test methods, resulting in improper treatment of patients if reported as RIF R instead of RIF susceptible [202, 289]. In other words, synonymous silent mutations detected as RS-TB by WGS, are potentially due to false-positive RIF R when LPA and/or Xpert results shows RR-TB. Thus, the results from this part of the study showed that the majority (76%) of synonymous silent mutations were among the *rpoB* small single nucleotide variants (SNVs), suggestive of potential false-positive RIF R. In support of the study findings in Chapter six, reports of false-positive RIF R results by Xpert/LPA were reported as the most likely cause of discrepancies between genotypic and phenotypic testing [290, 291]. Another study identified specimens that were RIF R with Xpert, but RIF susceptible with pDST and *rpoB* sequencing [292]. Additional reasons for possible false-positive RIF R results could be due to Xpert parameters; information on which is unfortunately limited in this part of the study and could not be investigated further. Yet, these parameters would include; i) probe delay where the delta cycle threshold (ΔCt) max value is between 4.1 and 4.9; ii) double probe delay (specifically delayed hybridization of probes D and E) and; iii) an abnormal graph fluorescence curve [293-295]. Lastly, false-positive RIF R results by Xpert could also occur when the *M.tb* bacterial load is very low (Ct > 28); thus, leading to discordant results [293, 294, 296]. To avoid false-positive RIF R by rapid diagnostic methods (Xpert/LPA), it is highly recommended that DNA sequencing or WGS (if available) is performed to predict resistance [294].

Certainly, one can also not overlook other possibilities for the above-mentioned discordance that were not anticipated, and could not be further explored in this study. These may have ranged from pre-analytic, analytic and post-analytic errors that are quite diverse and difficult to interpret [285]. Among these could include laboratory specimen mix-up or contamination. Also, it is possible that different sputum specimens used for initial molecular diagnostic *M.tb* testing could lead to different results. For instance, the first sputum specimen is utilized for Xpert testing, whereas subsequent LPA testing performed from cultured isolates utilizes the second sputum specimen. This may be due to heterogeneity of the examined sputum specimen and detection of genetically different strains that might come from separate lesions of the lungs that contain diverse *M.tb* strains that open simultaneously [274, 275, 277, 297, 298].

Discordance between phenotypic and genotypic DST may also be due to other mechanisms of RIF R that are not conferred by mutations, such as decreased cell penetrability to drugs and active efflux pumps [299, 300]. An efflux pump mechanism may be responsible for the ~5% RR-TB strains with no mutations detected in the RIF R determining region (RRDR). Both target gene mutations and efflux pumps are associated with resistance to anti-TB drugs. Through transcription-level analysis, Pang *et al.* [25] found that three efflux pumps where responsible in exporting RIF from its cell among RMR-TB isolates that were initially identified as RMR-TB without *rpoB* mutations with DNA sequencing. Furthermore, Li *et al.* [301] suggest that mutations in the *rpoB* gene, together with the identification of six specific putative efflux pump genes may have contributed to RMR-TB among RR-TB strains. Hence, more studies are needed to support these findings. Lastly, there could also be undefined and rarely reported *rpoB* mutations that are still unknown, and therefore not included in, for nstance, the database utilised by TB Profiler, and might be detected using targeted deep sequencing.

The second finding in this study was the significant difference in the proportion of high/moderate vs minimal confidence levels for *rpoB* mutations between RMR- and MDR-TB; with more high/moderate confidence *rpoB* mutations found among MDR-TB; demonstrating a strong association of those mutations with RIF R. The most predominant mutation found among MDR-TB was *rpoB* S531L (70%). S531L and *rpoB* mutations in codons 516 and 526 are commonly shown to confer high level RIF R, comprising 90% or more among phenotypic RIF R isolates in several studies globally [24, 26, 28, 278, 302-306]. On the other hand, two rarely reported *rpoB* mutations (T481A and V146F) that are found outside of the *rpoB* rifampicin resistance determining region (RRDR); that are not classified by Miotto *et al.* [147]; were identified by WGS TB profiler (RIF MIC 10-20 µg/ml - MGIT) in this study (Chapter six). Phelan *et al.* [307] found *rpoB* V146F (V170F) in only one isolate in their database that was identified as an interesting single nucleotide polymorphism (SNP) due to its closeness to the docked rifampicin ligand in their homology model; with the use of WGS and protein structure modelling. Also, Jamieson *et al.* [28] identified *rpoB* V146F with WGS among two MDR-TB isolates as a RIF R nonsynonymous mutation, with a RIF MIC of 50 µg/ml and a rifabutin MIC of 1 µg/ml (MGIT). Lastly, WGS tools PhyResSE and TBprofiler identified a double mutation T481A (T400A) and S531L in the same population, referring to them as heteroresistance [308]. Nonetheless, these mutations (T481A and V146F) seem to be of rare occurance and often not reported.

Lastly, this study found a statistically significant difference between RMR-TB and the presence of the *rpoB* L511P mutation compared to MDR-TB strains. L511P is described as a disputed mutation conferring minimal confidence or low-level RIF R [27, 147]. Notably, all 10 *rpoB* L511P strains (8 RMR-TB; 2 MDR-TB) tested phenotypically susceptible to RIF (RS-TB) with the MGIT q pDST; causing discrepancies between WGS and q pDST results. RIF MICs for *rpoB* L511P were found to be nearly four to ten times (≤0.125 µg/ml to 0.25 µg/ml) below the standard critical concentration (CC) of ≤1 µg/ml. The remaining L511P mutations from this study, also had RIF MICs of 0.5 µg/ml and 1 µg/ml, resulting in RS-TB with the MGIT. Moreover, WGS-derived results showed that all RMR-TB strains (n=46); including L511P; had no other mutations conferring resistance to any of the other TB drugs.

In support of the study findings from Chapter six of this book, *rpoB* L511P was found to significantly contribute to discrepancies between RR-TB strains (on Xpert) that tested RS-TB (on MGIT) from a study in Baku, Azerbaijan [306]. Furthermore, the findings from Chapter six within this book, are in concordance to many other studies that found *rpoB* L511P; as well as a few other disputed *rpoB* mutations (D516Y, H526N, H526L, H526S, L533P, I572F); causing discrepancies between genotypic and phenotypic MGIT pDST [24, 26, 31, 309-312]. However, not all disputed mutations confer low-level resistance, and the level of resistance is dependent on the type of disputed mutation. Previous studies have described that RIF MIC determination strongly relates to the position and the nature of the amino-acid substitution in the *rpoB* RRDR [313, 314]. In the past, the occurrence of disputed *rpoB* mutations were extremely rare [18]. However, studies now show that their occurrence are becoming more frequent and suggest that they may contribute to RIF R [27, 310, 315]. We suspect the reason for this rapid increase was since the introduction of Xpert for the initial diagnosis of screening RIF R in all patients in many settings; and not pDST (used prior to Xpert and LPA) for *M.tb* patients considered as high risk DR-TB patients. Van Deun *et al.* [31] found disputed *rpoB* mutations among 13.1% and 10.6% of all previously treated RR-TB patients from Bangladesh and Kinshasa, respectively. Furthermore, there have been reports of disputed mutations from RR-TB strains isolated from new TB patients [27, 316]. Miotto *et al.* [317] found disputed mutations (L511P, D516Y, H526L/N and L533P) that tested rifampicin susceptible on the MGIT ranging from 15% to 57% (overall 16/55 isolates). These authors confirm that disputed mutations are associated with growth impairment in MGIT rifampicin q pDST.

Moreover, evidence that the presence of L511P disputed mutations results in MICs four to ten times below the RIF standard CC with the MGIT, was reported in many studies [28, 96, 202, 318]. A previous study suggested that disputed mutations be confirmed using the proportion method in solid medium [31]; however, Jamieson *et al.* [28] found these mutations susceptible in both liquid MGIT and solid media. Van Deun *et al.* [24] previously reported that with liquid culture MGIT pDST, disputed mutations are found susceptible or are easily missed. Additional evidence shows that with solid culture pDST, these mutations confer low-level RIF R with minimal confidence [147]. These low-level RIF R isolates are difficult to detect because of fitness loss and slower growth in the presence of the RIF drug compared to the drug free controls [319], and might explain why RS-TB was reported on the MGIT and RR-TB by Xpert and/or LPA in this study (Chapter six). Briefly, even though these disputed mutations show rifampicin susceptibility with the MGIT pDST, low-level RIF resistance is still found on solid culture pDST; which is crucial information for clinicians to be made aware of in terms of TB treatment for patients. Furthermore, Rigouts *et al.* [26] suggested that the gold standard for rifampicin resistance should be reconsidered in order to address discordance between genotypic and phenotypic results. Other studies questioned the clinical relevance of the current RIF CC and suggest adjusting the CC used to define RIF R from the currently used 1 µg/ml to 0.5 µg/ml, or even as low as 0.0625 µg/ml

[28, 31, 275, 320, 321]. Briefly, this would change the susceptibility status of discrepant cases from "susceptible" to "resistant" in various studies (including this book research study). Additionally, pharmacokinetic/pharmacodynamics modelling of MIC data could help determine susceptibility breakpoints, especially for low-level resistant isolates [322, 323]. However, the clinical relevance of low-level RIF resistance and/or the presence of these disputed *rpoB* mutations is as yet unknown.

There is evidence that clinical diagnosis and decisions on TB treatment are often made by using a combination of phenotypic and genotypic test results [31, 324, 325]. In 2015, the WHO recommended that any patient with RR-TB; including RMR-TB patients; should be treated with an MDR-TB treatment regimen. Thus, RMR-TB patients with low-level RIF R are treated with a lengthy, more toxic MDR-TB regimen, implying that despite low-level RIF resistant mutations, standard regimens may not be effective. Since *rpoB* L511P was frequently found among RMR-TB strains in Khayelitsha, it does raise concerns with regards to TB treatment regimens used for low-level RIF resistance. Possible treatment could be higher drug doses for RIF [326, 327]; however, there could be other *in vivo* factors affecting clinical outcomes such as the *M.tb* strain population structure [328, 329], pharmacokinetic/ pharmacodynamic parameters [320], permeability of *M.tb* lesions and adverse reactions [330]. Gumbo *et al.* [331] suggested that higher doses of RIF may be efficacious in both improving bactericidal activity of RIF and preventing the emergence of RIF R isolates. These authors mentioned that assessing RIF efficacy, by the most relevant pharmacodynamic parameter is the ratio of area under the concentration-time curve (AUC) over the MIC (AUC/MIC) [331]. A study by, van Ingen *et al.* [327] evaluated AUC/MIC ratios in four patients with A516Y mutations with MICs up to 1 µg/ml, and suggested that high doses of RIF (20 mg/kg) could be sufficient to overcome low-level resistance. Since there have been reports of disputed mutations or low-level RIF resistance resulting in poor treatment outcomes in patients [27, 31, 327], substitution of rifampicin with rifabutin has also been suggested as an alternative to higher drug doses for RIF [332, 333]. Studies have shown that rifabutin positively affects the treatment outcome in patients with low-level RIF resistance [28, 333, 334]. However, the optimal duration for rifabutin-based regimens still needs further investigation [327].

In general, mutation frequencies in *rpoB* codon 511 were found to differ in various geographic settings globally, with ranges from 0% to 9.4% among RR-TB [335]. However, in South Korea, *rpoB* disputed mutations were identified in 11% (32/300) RR-TB strains, with L511P constituting 25% (8/32) of the strains [315]. In China, during April to December 2007, RIF susceptible isolates performed on solid culture qDST underwent further testing for *rpoB* mutations [336]. Findings revealed that 99% (3045/3077) of the strains had no *rpoB* mutations (RS-TB), while only 1% (32/3077) had *rpoB* mutations (RR-TB). Among the 32 strains with *rpoB* mutations, 31 were single mutations and one had a double mutation (L511P/H526G). Furthermore, L511P was found among 32% (10/31) of the strains with single mutations. Unfortunately, data on RMR- and MDR-TB strains were not available [336]. During 2009 to 2014, 7094 *M.tb* patients (6124 RS-TB; 970 RR-TB) were enrolled in a population-level survey performed in hospitals and clinics in seven countries globally (Azerbaijan, Bangledesh, Belarus, Pakistan, Phillippines, South Africa [Gauteng and Kwazulu Natal province] and Ukraine) [32]. The methods conducted included phenotypic DST (MGIT or LJ), as well as sequencing data obtained either through WGS or targeted gene sequencing. Also, mutations were considered as conferring RIF R when classified as either high, moderate or minimal confidence categories [147]. Results obtained showed that 4% (38/958) of RR-TB isolates had the L511P mutation. Among these strains with the L511P mutation, 20/38 (53%) tested phenotypically susceptible, whereas 18/38 (47%) tested phenotypically resistant; of which 10/18 were minimal confidence, and 8/18 were double *rpoB* mutations (L511P with either minimal (5/18), moderate (1/18) or high confidence (2/18) mutations. Notably, these results were obtained either from liquid MGIT or solid LJ medium without reporting specific MIC levels. Unfortunately, data on the relative prevalence of L511P across RMR- and MDR-TB isolates, and across countries was not available [32].

Several limitations are noted in this part of the study. Firstly, additional data could not be gathered for the Xpert or LPA results of mutations detected for RR-TB cases, as the NHLS data was not available before August 2015. Therefore, comparison of the initial reports on Xpert and/or verification of the initial LPA strip results to WGS mutation data, was not possible. Secondly, q pDST was performed using only the BACTEC MGIT 960 system, and not the solid agar proportion method, which may have been more sensitive in detecting low-level RIF R [24]. However, the current gold standard is the more rapid MGIT DST method due to the importance of timely diagnosis of DR-TB (usually 10-14 days) compared to 4-6 weeks after culture with solid agar DST [96]. It is therefore important to reassess the critical concentration across all utilised methods of phenotypic DST. Also, the MIC concentrations of high confidence level *rpoB* mutations were not measured, as there are already significant data available. Thirdly, discordance was not further explored with regard to WGS with no *rpoB* mutations (RS-TB), by additionally performing Sanger sequencing to confirm the absence or presence of RIF and INH related mutations (on both the MGIT and DNA extracted tubes sent for WGS); to further verify possible discordance. Furthermore, it is important to note that a larger subset of strains, over a longer time period, would give better insight of this topic in the setting of Khayelitsha. Nevertheless, this study investigated a broad overview of *rpoB* mutations circulating in Khayelitsha during 2013 to 2015; and provides linkage of clinical data at an individual patient level to WGS data of patient isolates in a high burden HIV and DR-TB setting. Notably, the availability of patient samples may not be a complete reflection of RR-TB burden in Khayelitsha during 2013 to 2015, due to the fact that not all strains from patient samples were stored and not all WGS data were available for further analysis.

## 7.2 Conclusion

As shown from this part of the study, we cannot ignore the fact that low-level RIF R; particularly *rpoB* L511P; is one of the most predominant strains circulating among RMR-TB patients in Khayelitsha, that is often not detected by the gold standard pDST; thus, with potentially significant implications for the treatment and clinical care of RR-TB patients. However, these low-level *rpoB* mutations are easily detected by WGS; readily identifying mutation types; which should preferably be used in conjunction with MIC testing for individualised patient treatment regimens, in order to accurately diagnosis RR-TB [144, 145, 337]. However, WGS is not routinely available in resource-limited settings where HIV and DR-TB burden is often the highest. Furthermore, discordance between genotypic and phenotypic testing, resulting from mixed infections and/or false-positive RIF R, may cause confusion for clinicians and can lead to possible misdiagnosis or mismanagement, resulting in poor treatment outcomes among patients. For instance, a patient with false-positive RIF R would be treated with an MDR-TB treatment regimen when the patient truly has RS-TB; and so forth. Nonetheless, we are hopeful that in future, direct WGS of *M.tb* isolated directly from specimens may assist in determining low-level RIF R, heteroresistance and/or false-positive RIF R, with an added benefit of identifying SNVs (identifying silent mutations); for better diagnosis of RIF R.

Currently, there are no clinical trial data on how to treat RMR-TB patients with low-level RIF R. Since there has been reports of disputed mutations or low-level RIF R resulting in poor clinical outcomes; [27, 31, 273, 316, 327, 338] higher doses of RIF [327], or substitution with rifabutin [332, 333] has been suggested for treatment. However, higher doses of RIF has not been investigated in terms of clinical outcomes, and the optimal duration for rifabutin-based regimens also needs further investigation [327]. Optimal drug regimens, especially for low-level and discordant RR-TB are currently undefined. Future research, focusing on WGS implementation and clinical management thereof, as well as economic benefits and constraints in various geographical settings, would be beneficial and is urgently needed for better diagnosis of RR-TB.

# CHAPTER EIGHT

# 8. Transmission cluster analysis (Results)

## 8.1 General overview

Among the 670 rifampicin-resistant TB (RR-TB) patients that were routinely diagnosed during 2013 to 2015 (inclusive), a total of 203 (30%) whole genome sequencing (WGS) derived RR-TB strains were available for further transmission analysis. For the analysis of recent transmission, parameters used within the pipeline in this study, were commonly used among other TB genomic researchers (refer to Chapter 3; section 3.11) [120, 210]. Thus, the inclusion of 203 genomes were derived from sputum samples taken from stored pre-treatment isolates [179/224 (80%)]; as well as stored isolates from patient sputum samples taken ≤ 30 days into TB treatment [24/39 (62%)] (Figure 8.1). The reason for these inclusions were based on the World Health Organization (WHO) definition of new TB cases to capture recent transmission [3].

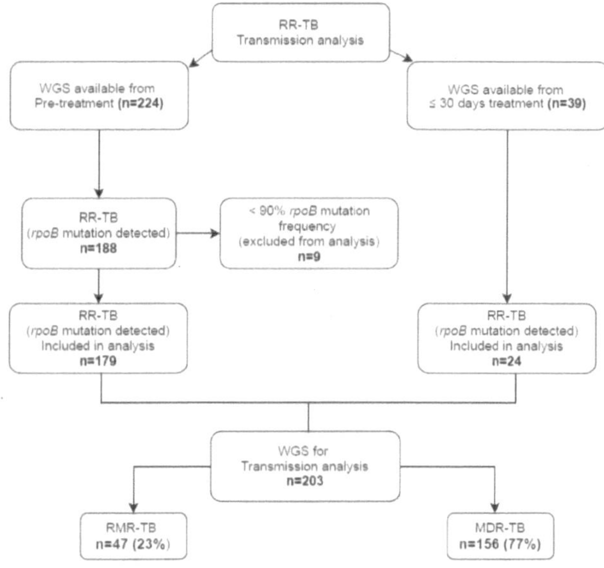


**Figure 8. 1** A flow diagram showing WGS-derived RR-TB strains for transmission analysis from RR-TB patients routinely diagnosed during 2013-15

To assess the potential for bias, demographic and clinical data were compared among patients where WGS data was available and not available during 2013 to 2015 (Table 8.1). Patients with WGS data available were more likely to have their previous TB treatment status known, less likely to have RR-TB just diagnosed with GeneXpert MTB/RIF (Xpert) only, and more likely to have had second-line treatment started (Table 8.1).

**Table 8. 1** Epidemiological comparison between WGS data not available (n=467) and WGS data available (n=203) for transmission cluster analysis among 670 routinely diagnosed RR-TB patients during 2013-15

| | **No WGS data available n=467 (%)** | **WGS data available n=203 (%)** | ***p-value* *** |
|---|---|---|---|
| ***Demographic & Clinical data*** | | | |
| Gender (Male) | 222 (48%) | 103 (51%) | *0.447* |
| (Female) | 245 (53%) | 100 (49%) | |
| Age (0-15) | 19 (4%) | 1 (1%) | *0.172* |
| (16-24) | 56 (12%) | 27 (13%) | |
| (25-34) | 163 (35%) | 74 (36%) | |
| (35-44) | 137 (29%) | 63 (31%) | |
| (45-54) | 64 (14%) | 30 (15%) | |
| (55+) | 28 (6%) | 8 (4%) | |
| HIV status known | 461 (99%) | 203 (100%) | *0.109* |
| HIV positive among known | 355 (76%) | 155 (76%) | *0.530* |
| Previous TB treatment known | 450 (96%) | 203 (100%) | ***0.001*** |
| Previously treated among known | 278 (60%) | 124 (61%) | *0.708* |
| ***RR-TB profile (according to routinely diagnosed results)*** | | | |
| GeneXpert unconfirmed/discordant RR-TB | 71 (15%) | 0 | ***<0.001*** |
| RMR-TB (among those with RIF & INH DST) | 101 (26%) | 49 (24%) | *0.473* |
| MDR-TB (among those with RIF and INH DST) | 295 (74%) | 154 (76%) | *0.719* |
| RR-TB treatment started | 404 (87%) | 201 (99%) | ***<0.001*** |

*Chi-squared for difference in proportions

## 8.2 Strain diversity

Rifampicin mono-resistant TB (RMR-TB) strains mainly comprised of Lineage 4 (Euro-American; S type) (Figure 8.2). In contrast, among the multi-drug resistant TB (MDR-TB) strains, Lineage 2 (East Asian; Beijing) was predominantly found, followed by Lineage 4 (Euro-American; LAM) (Table 8.2; Figure 8.2). The proportion of Lineage 2 strains between RMR-TB (36%) and MDR-TB (72%) was significantly different (p<0.001) (Table 8.2).

**Table 8. 2** Global genome-based phylogeny of RMR- and MDR-TB strain lineages based on large sequence polymorphisms (LSP) and spoligotyping based families

| Genome-based phylogeny (Comas *et al.*) | LSP based lineages (Gagneux *et al.*) | Spoligotyping based families (Brudey *et al.*) | RMR-TB (n = 47) | MDR-TB (n = 156) | Total (n = 203) |
|---|---|---|---|---|---|
| Lineage 1 | Indo-Oceanic | EAI | 3 (6%) | 2 (1%) | 5 (2%) |
| Lineage 2 | East Asian | Beijing | 17 (36%) | 113 (72%) | 130 (64%) |
| Lineage 3 | East-African-Indian | CAS | 3 (6%) | 0 | 3 (1%) |
| Lineage 4 | Euro-American | LAM, Haarlem, S-type, mainly T, X-type, H37Rv | 24 (51%) | 41 (26%) | 65 (32%) |
| **Total** | | | ***47*** | ***156*** | ***203 * p<0.001*** |

*Chi-squared for difference in proportions
**Definitions:** EAI (East-African-Indian); CAS (Central Asian); LAM (Latin American Mediterranean)
**Note:** 'East African Indian' and EAI spoligotype family refer to completely different strain lineages
**References:** Comas *et al.* [339]; Gagneux *et al.* [117]; Brudey *et al.* [108]

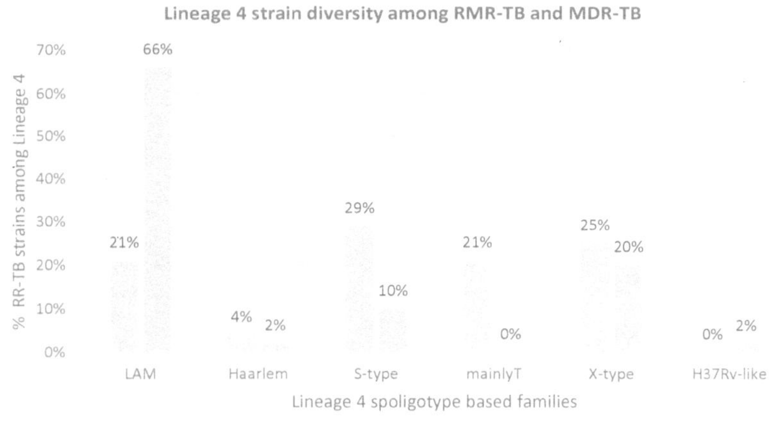


**Figure 8. 2** Strain diversity found among Lineage 4, RMR-TB and MDR-TB strains

## 8.3 Transmission cluster analysis

Clusters identified with Clusterpicker and the single nucleotide polymorphism (SNP) distance matrix (SNP differences found between genomes), were correlated when a SNP threshold of 12 was used. A total number of 121/203 (60%) clustered strains were found (Tables 8.3 and 8.4), resulting in 35 genomic clusters (Tables 8.5 to 8.7). Figure 8.3 shows a phylogenetic tree indicating the genomic clusters and lineages; highlighted in groups of colours on the periphery, as well as branches. The largest cluster group were MDR-TB strains (n=15, lineage 2), all of which had *rpoB* S531L mutations. However, most genomic clusters (19/35; 54%) contained only two strains (Table 8.5).

A significant difference in clustering was found between RMR- and MDR-TB strains; with more MDR-TB isolates clustered, suggesting a greater contribution of recent transmission to the disease burden ($p<0.001$) (Table 8.3). More clustering was found among lineage 2 (93/130; 72%) compared to lineage 4 (26/65; 40%) among all RR-TB, including RMR- and MDR-TB ($p<0.001$). In total, seven clusters were identified among RMR-TB strains (17 of 47 isolates; 36%) (Table 8.5).

**Table 8. 3** The number of clustered and non-clustered RR-TB strains according to WGS

| WGS-based | RMR-TB (n = 47) | All MDR-TB regardless of SL resistance (n = 156) | Total (n=203) |
|---|---|---|---|
| Clustered | 17 (36%) | 104 (67%) | 121 |
| Non-clustered | 30 (64%) | 52 (33%) | 82 |
| ***Total*** | ***47*** | ***156*** | ***203*** *p<0.001* |

**Note:** SL refers to Second-line

**Table 8. 4** Detailed summary of RR-TB profile of clustered strains according to WGS

| RR-TB profile (WGS-based) | No. of strains (n=203) | No. of strains clustered (n=121) |
|---|---|---|
| RMR-TB | 47 | 17 (36%) |
| All MDR-TB | 156 | 104 (67%) |
| ➢ *MDR-TB* | *108* | *66 (61%)* |
| ➢ *preXDR FLQ* | *7* | *6 (86%)* |
| ➢ *preXDR INJ* | *25* | *19 (76%)* |
| ➢ *XDR-TB* | *16* | *13 (81%)* |

**Table 8. 5** Detailed table showing *rpoB* mutations and strain lineages found among RMR- and MDR-TB genomic clusters within a SNP threshold of 12

| WGS genomic clusters | No. of strains per cluster | Study number per strain | WGS strain lineage | WGS drug class | *rpoB* mutations | *rpoB* confidence level |
|---|---|---|---|---|---|---|
| **1** | **4** | **[TB47, TB53, TB88, TB191]** | **L4 (S-type)** | **RMR** | **D516F** | **high** |
| 2 | 9 | [TB164, TB110, TB39, TB159, TB59, TB207, TB48, TB129, TB121] | L4 (LAM) | MDR | S531L | high |
| **3** | **2** | **[TB174, TB6]** | **L3 (CAS)** | **RMR** | **S531L** | **high** |
| 4 | 4 | [TB12, TB160, TB176, TB195] | L4 (LAM) | MDR | S531L | high |
| **5** | **3** | **[TB199, TB8, TB198]** | **L4 (X-type)** | **RMR** | **L511P** | **minimal** |
| 6 | 2 | [TB70, TB190] | L4 (LAM) | MDR | S531L | high |
| 7 | 2 | [TB206, TB197] | L4 (X-type) | MDR | S531L | high |
| 8 | 2 | [TB149, TB76] | L4 (X-type) | MDR | D516V | high |
| 9 | 2 | [TB186, TB196] | L2 (Beijing) | MDR | L533P | moderate |
| 10 | 2 | [TB124, TB163] | L2 (Beijing) | MDR | S531L | high |
| 11 | 4 | [TB38, TB220, TB25, TB20] | L2 (Beijing) | MDR | D516V | high |
| 12 | 3 | [TB178, TB2, TB194] | L2 (Beijing) | MDR | S531L | high |
| 13 | 3 | [TB101, TB82, TB90] | L2 (Beijing) | MDR | S531L | high |
| 14 | 2 | [TB46, TB204] | L2 (Beijing) | MDR | S531L | high |
| **15** | **2** | **[TB56, TB69]** | **L2 (Beijing)** | **RMR** | **H526Y** | **high** |
| 16 | 2 | [TB75, TB212] | L2 (Beijing) | MDR | D516V | high |
| 17 | 3 | [TB202, TB161, TB214] | L2 (Beijing) | MDR | D516V | high |
| 18 | 2 | [TB87, TB123] | L2 (Beijing) | MDR | S531L | high |
| 19 | 7 | [TB208, TB188, TB117, TB134, TB96, TB150, TB192] | L2 (Beijing) | MDR | H526Y | high |
| 20 | 2 | [TB133, TB187] | L2 (Beijing) | MDR | S531L | high |
| **21** | **2** | **[TB105, TB34]** | **L2 (Beijing)** | **RMR** | **L511P** | **minimal** |
| 22 | 2 | [TB135, TB31] | L2 (Beijing) | MDR | S531L | high |
| 23 | 2 | [TB128, TB210] | L2 (Beijing) | MDR | S531L | high |
| **24** | **2** | **[TB122, TB65]** | **L2 (Beijing)** | **RMR** | **H526Y** | **high** |
| 25 | 2 | [TB155, TB102] | L2 (Beijing) | MDR | H526N<br>L533P | minimal<br>moderate |
| **26** | **2** | **[TB66, TB60]** | **L2 (Beijing)** | **RMR** | **H526D** | **high** |
| 27 | 5 | [TB86, TB116, TB218, TB158, TB130] | L2 (Beijing) | MDR | S531L | high |
| 28 | 2 | [TB103, TB173] | L2 (Beijing) | MDR | S531L | high |
| 29 | 3 | [TB19, TB145, TB213] | L2 (Beijing) | MDR | S531L | high |
| 30 | 4 | [TB98, TB166, TB1, TB181] | L2 (Beijing) | MDR | S531L | high |
| 31 | 6 | [TB147, TB77, TB92, TB170, TB68, TB132] | L2 (Beijing) | MDR | S531L | high |
| 32 | 15 | [TB209, TB141, TB211, TB118, TB193, TB37, TB115, TB136, TB216, TB140, TB78, TB14, TB127, TB99, TB144] | L2 (Beijing) | MDR | S531L | high |
| 33 | 7 | [TB177, TB41, TB15, TB28, TB119, TB137, TB146] | L2 (Beijing) | MDR | S531L | high |
| 34 | 3 | [TB51, TB219, TB97] | L2 (Beijing) | MDR | S531L | high |
| 35 | 2 | [TB112, TB5] | L2 (Beijing) | MDR | S531L | high |

**Note:** RMR-TB genomic clusters are highlighted in bold. Refer to Figure 8.3 to view the phylogenetic tree

**Table 8. 6** A summarized table of WGS clustered genomic strains among all RR-TB

| No. of strains per cluster | Total no. of clusters | Total no. of strains in all clusters |
|---|---|---|
| 2 | 19 (54%) | 38 (31%) |
| 3 | 6 (17%) | 18 (15%) |
| 4 | 4 (11%) | 16 (13%) |
| 5 | 1 (3%) | 5 (4%) |
| 6 | 1 (3%) | 6 (5%) |
| 7 | 2 (6%) | 14 (13%) |
| 9 | 1 (3%) | 9 (7%) |
| 15 | 1 (3%) | 15 (12%) |
| ***Total*** | ***35*** | ***121*** |

**Table 8. 7** A summarized table of WGS clustered genomic strains among RMR- and MDR-TB

| | **RMR-TB** | | **MDR-TB** | |
|---|---|---|---|---|
| No. of strains per cluster | Total no. of cluster groups | Total no. of strains in all cluster groups | Total no. of cluster groups | Total no. of strains in all cluster groups |
| 2 | 5 | 10 | 14 | 28 |
| 3 | 1 | 3 | 5 | 15 |
| 4 | 1 | 4 | 3 | 12 |
| 5 | 0 | 0 | 1 | 5 |
| 6 | 0 | 0 | 1 | 6 |
| 7 | 0 | 0 | 2 | 14 |
| 9 | 0 | 0 | 1 | 9 |
| 15 | 0 | 0 | 1 | 15 |
| ***Total*** | ***7*** | ***17*** | ***28*** | ***104*** |

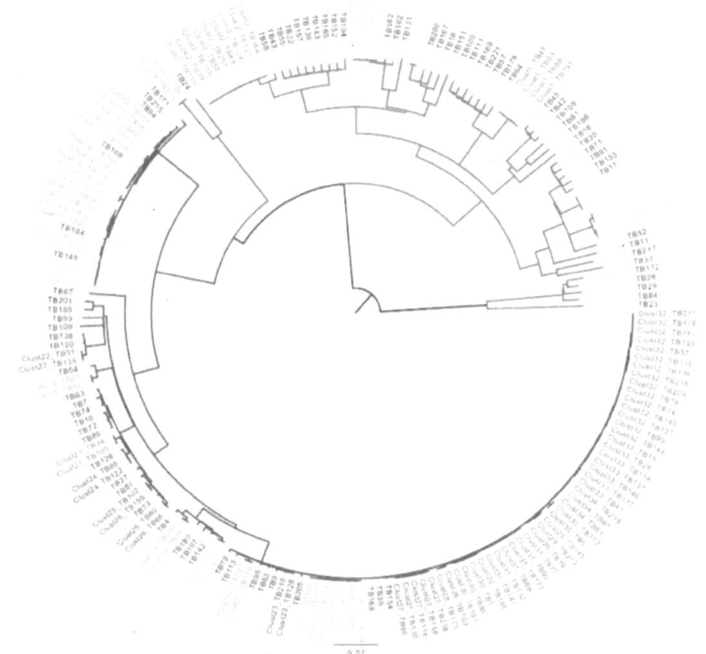

Pink branch = L1 (EAI); Indo Oceanic
Blue branch = L2 (Beijing); East Asian
Purple branch = L3 (CAS); East African Indi
Red branch = L4 (LAM & others); Euro-Am

SNP threshold of 12

**Figure 8. 3** Phylogenetic tree showing WGS transmission clusters found among RR-TB strains during 2013-15 in Khayelitsha

**Note:** Clustered groups are highlighted in various colours along the periphery e.g Clust35_TB5 (Refer to Table 8.5). Genomes not clustered are in black text e.g TB180.

When looking at the results from the 203 WGS data that were available, no significant differences were found in clustering by HIV status and previous TB treatment history among all RR-TB, including RMR- and MDR-TB (Table 8.8; Table 8.9).

**Table 8. 8** Clustering among all RR-TB stratified by HIV status and previous TB treatment history

| | No. of RR-TB strains | Clustered (%) |
|---|---|---|
| ***HIV status*** | | |
| HIV positive | 155 | 90/155 (58%) |
| HIV negative | 48 | 31/48 (65%) |
| ***Total*** | ***203*** | ***121/203 (60%)*** *p=0.688* |
| ***Previous TB treatment history*** | | |
| Previously treated | 124 | 76/124 (61%) |
| No previous treatment (new) | 79 | 45/79 (57%) |
| ***Total*** | ***203*** | ***121/203 (60%)*** *p=0.761* |

**Table 8. 9** Clustering among RMR- and MDR-TB stratified by HIV status and previous TB treatment history

| | RMR-TB | | MDR-TB | |
|---|---|---|---|---|
| | N | Clustered (%) | N | Clustered (%) |
| ***HIV status*** | | | | |
| HIV positive | 36 | 12/36 (33%) | 119 | 78/119 (66%) |
| HIV negative | 11 | 5/11 (45%) | 37 | 26/37 (70%) |
| ***Total*** | ***47*** | ***17/47 (36%)*** | ***156*** | ***67/156 (43%)*** *p=0.692* |
| ***Previous TB treatment history*** | | | | |
| Previously treated | 31 | 12/31 (39%) | 93 | 64/93 (69%) |
| No previous treatment (new) | 16 | 5/16 (31%) | 63 | 40/63 (63%) |
| ***Total*** | ***47*** | ***17 (36%)*** | ***156*** | ***67/156 (43%)*** *p=0.496* |

Furthermore, we found that RR-TB was due to direct transmission in 63% (128/203) of the patients (Figure 8.4). From a total of 35 genomic clusters, three of them (clusters 20, 22, 34) all included patients who were treatment naïve.

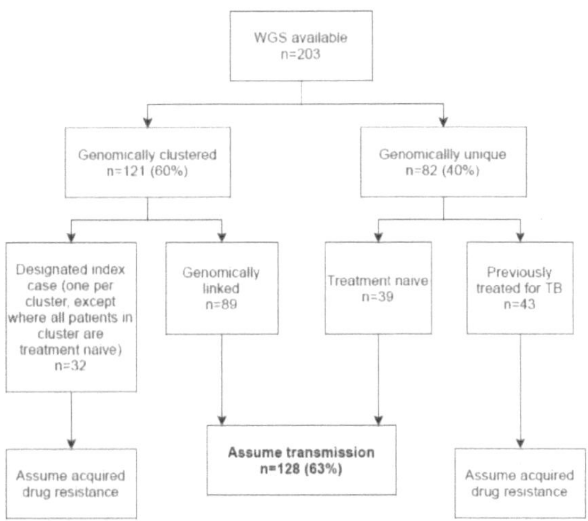


**Figure 8. 4** Clustered versus unique genomes to illustrate suggestive direct transmission among 203 WGS data available for transmission cluster analysis during 2013-15

Moreover, more isolates with WGS data were available from 2015 (Table 8.10). Although numbers are small, among the 113 MDR-TB strains with *rpoB* S531L mutation, 73% clustered compared to 17% among the 12 RMR-TB strains with the same S531L mutation (Table 8.11). On the other hand, among the 10 RMR-TB strains with *rpoB* L511P mutation, 50% clustered whereas no clustering was found among MDR-TB strains (although only two strains) with the same L511P mutation (Table 8.11). All health care facilities and clinics located in Khayelitsha are illustrated in Table 8.12 and Figure 8.5.

**Table 8. 10** Epidemiological comparison between all RR-TB diagnosed (n=670) and WGS data available (n=203) for transmission cluster analysis during 2013-15

| Year of diagnosis | All RR-TB diagnosed (% of total) | WGS data available (% of all RR-TB) | p-value |
|---|---|---|---|
| 2013 | 218 (32%) | 68/218 (31%) | |
| 2014 | 240 (36%) | 53/240 (26%) | *0.018* |
| 2015 | 212 (32%) | 82/212 (39%) | |
| *Total* | *670* | *203* | |

**Table 8. 11** Representation of the total number of MDR-TB (156) and RMR-TB (47) *rpoB* mutations categorised by confidence levels that clustered (WGS-based)

| | **High/moderate confidence *rpoB* mutations** | | | **Minimal/low confidence *rpoB* mutations** | | |
|---|---|---|---|---|---|---|
| | ***rpoB* mutation** | **Total** | **Clustered n (%)** | ***rpoB* mutation** | **Total** | **Clustered n (%)** |
| **MDR-TB** | S531L | 113 | 82/113 (73%) | H526N | 2 | 1/2 (50%) |
| | D516V | 13 | 11/13 (85%) | I572F | 1 | 0 |
| | H525Y | 8 | 7/8 (88%) | L511P | 2 | 0 |
| | L533P | 3 | 3/3 (100%) | | | |
| | H526D | 5 | 0 | | | |
| | H526L | 2 | 0 | | | |
| | D516Y | 2 | 0 | | | |
| | Q531K | 2 | 0 | | | |
| | S531F | 1 | 0 | | | |
| | T481A * | 2 | 0 | | | |
| ***Total (MDR-TB)*** | | ***151*** | ***103*** | | ***5*** | ***1*** |
| **RMR-TB** | S531L | 12 | 2/12 (17%) | L511P | 10 | 5/10 (50%) |
| | H526Y | 11 | 4/11 (36%) | | | |
| | H526D | 3 | 2/3 (67%) | | | |
| | D516F | 4 | 4/4 (100%) | | | |
| | L533P | 2 | 0 | | | |
| | S522L | 2 | 0 | | | |
| | D516G | 1 | 0 | | | |
| | D516Y | 1 | 0 | | | |
| | H526L | 1 | 0 | | | |
| ***Total (RMR-TB)*** | | ***37*** | ***12*** | | ***10*** | ***5*** |

**rpoB* mutation not classified by Miotto *et al.* [147]

**Table 8. 12** The location of 11 health care facilities in Khayelitsha

| Health care facilities/clinics | Location in Khayelitsha |
|---|---|
| Khayelitsha day hospital (KDH) | Mandela Park |
| Michael Mapongwana | Harare |
| Kuyasa | Town 3 |
| Luvuyo | T3-V3 |
| Mayenzeke | T3-V3 |
| Matthew Goniwe | T3-V5 |
| Town 2 | Silver Town |
| Zakhele | Village 1 North |
| Site B | Village 2 North |
| Site B Youth | Village 2 North |
| Nolungile | Ikwezi Park |

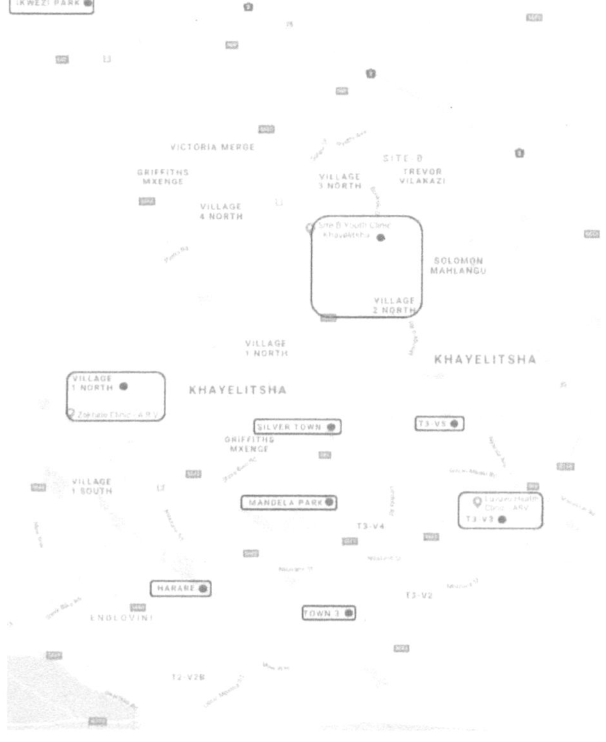


Adapted from: google maps

**Figure 8. 5** Maps illustrating the location of health care facilities and clinics in Khayelitsha

## 8.4 SNP differences among RMR-TB clusters

The following section includes detailed information regarding the clinical history and SNP differences from all genomic clusters found among RMR-TB patients only. Notably, all SNP differences were found within ~5 SNPs, even though a 12 SNP threshold was used.

### 8.4.1 Cluster 1 – Lineage 4 (*rpoB* D516F)

RMR-TB patients from cluster 1 were identified within lineage 4, Euro-American (S-type); with *rpoB* D516F (high confidence). All four patients were diagnosed in different clinics, were all HIV positive; while most of them (three patients) had received previous TB treatment. There were two males and two females with age ranges of 26 to 55 years old (Table 8.13). Although no connections were made to immediately link any of these patients, the SNP differences ranging from 1 to 6 is suggestive of transmission or a highly endemic strain (Table 8.14; Figure 8.6).

**Table 8. 13** Clinical information of RMR-TB patients within cluster 1

| | **Patient A** | **Patient B** | **Patient C** | **Patient D** |
|---|---|---|---|---|
| **Study ID** | TB88 | TB47 | TB53 | TB191 |
| **Clinic** | Clinic A | Clinic B | Clinic C | Clinic D |
| **Year of diagnoses** | 2013 | 2014 (6 months later than Patient A) | 2014 (8 months later than Patient B) | 2015 (5 months later than Patient C) |
| **HIV status** | Positive | Positive | Positive | Positive |
| **Previous TB treatment** | Yes | Yes | Yes | No |
| **Treatment outcomes** | Loss to follow-up | Completed treatment | Cured | Cured |

**Table 8. 14** SNP differences among RMR-TB patients within cluster 1

| **Study ID (Patient)** | TB191 **(Patient D)** | TB47 **(Patient B)** | TB53 **(Patient C)** | TB88 **(Patient A)** |
|---|---|---|---|---|
| TB191 **(D)** | **0** | 2 | 1 | 4 |
| TB47 **(B)** | | **0** | 1 | 6 |
| TB53 **(C)** | | | **0** | 5 |
| TB88 **(A)** | | | | **0** |

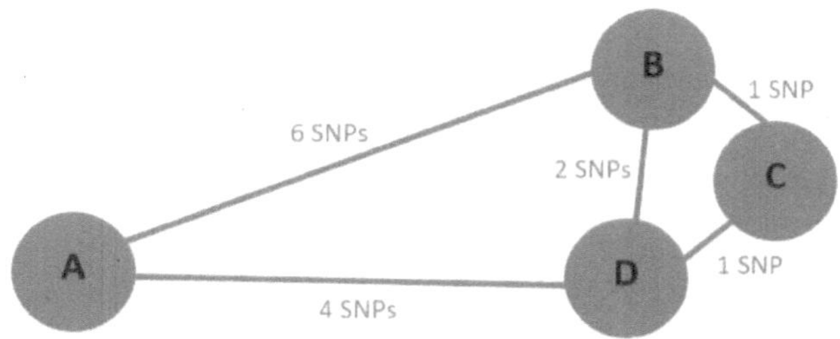


**Figure 8. 6** Minimum spanning tree for Cluster 1 to visually determine transmission among each genomic strain

**Note:** Branches indicate the number of unique SNPs between isolates with a 12 SNP threshold. Each number node corresponds to patients within Cluster 1.

### 8.4.2 Cluster 3 – Lineage 3 (*rpoB* S531L)

RMR-TB patients from cluster 3 were identified within lineage 3, East African Indian (CAS); with *rpoB* S531L (high confidence). Patient A was 28 years of age (female) and patient B was 41 years of age (male), and were diagnosed two years apart in different primary care clinics in Khayelitsha (Table 8.15). However, there was only a three SNP difference between these genomes, highly suggestive of transmission (Table 8.16).

**Table 8. 15** Clinical information of RMR-TB patients within cluster 3

| | **Patient A** | **Patient B** |
|---|---|---|
| **Clinic** | Clinic A | Clinic B |
| **Year of diagnoses** | 2013 | 2015 (2 years later than Patient A) |
| **HIV status** | Negative | Negative |
| **Previous TB treatment** | Yes | No |
| **Treatment outcomes** | Cured | Completed treatment |

**Table 8. 16** SNP differences among RMR-TB patients within cluster 3

| **Study ID (Patient)** | TB174 **(Patient B)** | TB6 **(Patient A)** |
|---|---|---|
| TB174 **(B)** | **0** | 3 |
| TB6 **(A)** | | **0** |

### 8.4.3 Cluster 5 – Lineage 4 (*rpoB* L511P)

RMR-TB patients from cluster 5 were identified within lineage 4, Euro-American (X-type); L511P (minimal confidence). All patients were HIV negative males, aged 27 to 40 years, and two were diagnosed in the same facility within the same year (two months apart) (Table 8.17). Given that only one SNP difference separated the genomes from these patients, the likelihood of these patients being involved in a direct chain of transmission is highly probable (Table 8.18).

Table 8. 17 Clinical information of RMR-TB patients within cluster 5

| | **Patient A** | **Patient B** | **Patient C** |
|---|---|---|---|
| **Clinic** | Clinic A | Clinic B | Clinic B |
| **Year of diagnoses** | 2013 | 2013<br>(2 months later than Patient A) | 2013<br>(2 months later than Patient B) |
| **HIV status** | Negative | Negative | Negative |
| **Previous TB treatment** | No | Yes | Yes |
| **Treatment outcomes** | Cured | Loss to follow-up | Died after being loss to follow-up |

Table 8. 18 SNP differences among RMR-TB patients within cluster 5

| **Study ID (Patient)** | TB198 **(Patient A)** | TB199 **(Patient C)** | TB8 **(Patient B)** |
|---|---|---|---|
| TB198 **(A)** | **0** | 1 | 0 |
| TB199 **(C)** | | **0** | 1 |
| TB8 **(B)** | | | **0** |

### 8.4.4 Cluster 15 – Lineage 2 (*rpoB* H526Y)

RMR-TB patients from cluster 15 were identified within lineage 2, East Asian (Beijing); with *rpoB* H526Y (high confidence). Both patients were female, aged 37 and 32 years, were HIV positive, and diagnosed in the same primary care clinic nine months apart (Table 8.19). These genomes were also identical, suggesting recent transmission (Table 8.20).

**Table 8. 19** Clinical information of RMR-TB patients within cluster 15

| | **Patient A** | **Patient B** |
|---|---|---|
| **Clinic** | Clinic A | Clinic A |
| **Year of diagnoses** | 2015 | 2015 (9 months later than Patient A) |
| **HIV status** | Positive | Positive |
| **Previous TB treatment** | Yes | No |
| **Treatment outcomes** | Died after being loss to follow-up | Cured |

**Table 8. 20** SNP differences among RMR-TB patients within cluster 15

| **Study ID (Patient)** | TB56 **(Patient A)** | TB69 **(Patient B)** |
|---|---|---|
| TB56 **(A)** | **0** | 0 |
| TB69 **(B)** | | **0** |

### 8.4.5 Cluster 21 – Lineage 2 (*rpoB* L511P)

RMR-TB patients from cluster 21 were identified within lineage 2, East Asian (Beijing); L511P (minimal confidence). Both patients were males, aged 37 and 44 years, diagnosed in different clinics in the same year (two months apart) (Table 8.21). SNP differences of five indicates transmission (Table 8.22).

**Table 8. 21** Clinical information of RMR-TB patients within cluster 21

| | **Patient A** | **Patient B** |
|---|---|---|
| **Clinic** | Clinic A | Clinic B |
| **Year of diagnoses** | 2013 | 2013 (2 months later than Patient A) |
| **HIV status** | Positive | Positive |
| **Previous TB treatment** | Yes | No |
| **Treatment outcomes** | Cured | Completed treatment |

**Table 8. 22** SNP differences among RMR-TB patients within cluster 21

| **Study ID (Patient)** | TB105 **(Patient A)** | TB34 **(Patient B)** |
|---|---|---|
| TB105 **(A)** | **0** | 5 |
| TB34 **(B)** | | **0** |

### 8.4.6 Cluster 24 – Lineage 2 (*rpoB* H526Y)

RMR-TB patients from cluster 24 were identified within lineage 2, East Asian (Beijing); H526Y (high confidence). Both HIV positive patients with a history of prior TB treatment were males, aged 32 and 30 years, diagnosed in different clinics (Table 8.23). SNP differences indicates transmission (Table 8.24).

**Table 8. 23** Clinical information of RMR-TB patients within cluster 24

| | **Patient A** | **Patient B** |
|---|---|---|
| **Clinic** | Clinic A | Clinic B |
| **Year of diagnoses** | 2014 | 2015 (7 months later than Patient A) |
| **HIV status** | Positive | Positive |
| **Previous TB treatment** | Yes | Yes |
| **Treatment outcomes** | Loss to follow-up | Completed treatment |

**Table 8. 24** SNP differences among RMR-TB patients within cluster 24

| **Study ID (Patient)** | TB122 **(Patient A)** | TB65 **(Patient B)** |
|---|---|---|
| TB122 **(A)** | **0** | 5 |
| TB65 **(B)** | | **0** |

### 8.4.7 Cluster 26 – Lineage 2 (*rpoB* H526D)

RMR-TB patients from cluster 26 were identified within lineage 2, East Asian (Beijing); H526D (high confidence). Patient A was female (33 years) and patient B was male (37 years). Both patients were diagnosed in different clinics and were HIV positive with a prior treatment history (Table 8.25). Thus, a SNP difference of one, as well as diagnoses within three months apart between these patients is highly suggestive of recent transmission (Table 8.26).

**Table 8. 25** Clinical information of RMR-TB patients within cluster 26

| | **Patient A** | **Patient B** |
|---|---|---|
| **Clinic** | Clinic A | Clinic B |
| **Year of diagnoses** | 2015 | 2015 (3 months later than Patient A) |
| **HIV status** | Positive | Positive |
| **Previous TB treatment** | Yes | Yes |
| **Treatment outcomes** | Cured | Loss to follow-up |

**Table 8. 26** SNP differences among RMR-TB patients within cluster 26

| **Study ID (Patient)** | TB60 **(Patient A)** | TB66 **(Patient B)** |
|---|---|---|
| TB60 **(A)** | **0** | 1 |
| TB66 **(B)** | | **0** |

# CHAPTER NINE

# 9. Transmission cluster analysis (Discussion

## 9.1 Discussion

This part of the study provides insights into the transmission of rifampicin-resistant TB (RR-TB) in Khayelitsha, including multi-drug resistant TB (MDR-TB) and rifampicin mono-resistant tuberculosis (RMR-TB) strains from whole genome sequencing (WGS) data that was available during 2013 to 2015. The key findings were that more clustering was found among MDR-TB compared to RMR-TB strains; specifically for *rpoB* S531L; suggesting that MDR-TB is more commonly due to direct transmission than RMR-TB. Moreover, Lineage 2 (L2) strains were more commonly found among MDR-TB compared to RMR-TB. Additionally, there was more clustering found among L2 compared to Lineage 4 (L4) among both MDR- and RMR-TB strains. Clustering among MDR- and RMR-TB differed when compared to high and minimal/low confidence *rpoB* mutations. Hence, among *rpoB* S531L (high confidence mutation) more MDR-TB strains (73%) clustered compared to RMR-TB (17%) strains. In contrast, among *rpoB* L511P (minimal/low confidence mutation) more RMR-TB strains (5/10; 50%) clustered compared to no clustering found among MDR-TB strains.

Many studies have shown that Beijing strains from L2 are widespread in different geographica settings, and occur more frequently in clusters with highly transmissible strains [151, 163, 340, 341]. In this part of the study, Beijing strains (L2) among MDR-TB, appeared to be endemic in Khayelitsha (during 2013-2015), as the high level of clustering suggests ongoing endemic spread. In addition, more clustering was found among MDR-TB *rpoB* S531L (high confidence mutation) compared to RMR-TB. Zignol *et al.* [32] reported *rpoB* S531L in 98% RR-TB strains among seven countries globally. Overall, evidence of this was also shown in several countries [26, 28, 278, 302-305]. In contrast, in Botswana there is evidence that the *M.tb* epidemic is dominated by L4 strains [342]; however clarity on RMR-TB strains is lacking. Similar to the results found in this book (Chapter eight), L2 strains have been reported in some countries with increased transmission [343, 344] and high MDR-TB prevalence [9]. Reports from African countries show a rapid increase in L2 [345-351] associated with drug resistance and transmission [41, 151, 352]. Rutaihwa *et al.* [353] investigated the evolutionary history of L2 in Africa. Their results illustrated that the introduction of L2 into Africa, during the past 300 years, was related to independent bacterial populations from East and Southeast Asia. Authors suggest that the success of L2 in Africa could be because of its high transmissibility and hypervirulence rather than drug resistance [353].

On the other hand, it appears as if RMR-TB is less transmissible than MDR-TB in this research study; despite the limited sample size reflecting only three years of data. Perhaps a larger study number, over a longer time period might portray a different story of RMR-TB transmission in Khayelitsha. With that said, RMR-TB transmission was mostly found among the following high confidence *rpoB* mutations, respectively, D516F, H526D/Y and S531L. However, although numbers are small, this study does show some degree of RMR-TB transmission among minimal/low confidence *rpoB* L511P mutation (5/10; 50%). Clinical information showed that the first RMR-TB L511P cluster with three HIV negative male patients were most likely due to closely related nosocomial transmission, as all three patients were diagnosed within two months apart at the same healthcare facility in Khayelitsha. Unfortunately, the last patient diagnosed within this cluster died after the treatment outcome of loss to follow-up. Notably, only one single nucleotide polymorphism (SNP) difference separated the genomes from these patients, likely indicating a direct chain of transmission. Previous studies have shown that genetic distances between strains, within a SNP distance of 0–5, confirmed epidemiological links between strains isolated from patients [63, 156, 157, 159, 160]. Thus, a SNP threshold of ≤5 has been suggested to indicate recent transmission [156, 161], whereas strains with >12 SNPs apart were not directly transmitted between patients. In addition, a systematic review published in 2016, provided confirmation of the above-mentioned from 12 studies [163]. In this part of the study (Chapter eight), the last RMR-TB L511P cluster with only two HIV positive male patients was most likely due to either closely related community acquired transmission, or nosocomial transmission (diagnosed two months apart at different healthcare facilities within Khayelitsha); with no evidence of household contacts in any of the above RMR-TB clusters. Also, a SNP difference of five suggested direct transmission between these patients.

As highlighted above, it is well known that drug-resistant TB (DR-TB) can spread efficiently through direct person to person transmission [35, 69]. Transmission of DR-TB can either occur between close contacts within households, hospitals/clinics or other settings. Other routes of transmission have been reported as individuals have casual contact at bars or restaurants, schools or workplaces, or the use of public transport in low incidence settings [67, 77]. For instance, in South Africa, KwaZulu Natal province, particularly in Msinga district, nosocomial transmission was a significant cause of MDR- and XDR-TB transmission [354]. Thus, this part of the study (Chapter eight) found that at least 63% of RR-TB (both MDR- and RMR-TB) was due to direct transmission in Khayelitsha during 2013-2015. Furthermore, this study (Chapter eight) did not find any differences in clustering by HIV status and previous TB treatment history among RMR- and MDR-TB patients (all RR-TB) when associated to the

203 WGS data that was available during 2013 to 2015. Multiple studies have shown that the majority of MDR-TB in endemic regions are due to transmission of already resistant strains rather than acquisition [35, 153, 355, 356]. While this may be true, evidence has also shown that patients previously exposed to rifampicin treatment are at greater risk of developing RR-TB [48, 357]. In addition to acquisition of DR-TB, studies have confirmed that patients with previous TB treatment history might be re-infected with a new DR-TB strain [57-59]. In settings with high HIV prevalence, it is possible that superinfection of DR-TB strains can occur with more than one TB strain [61, 62]. A mixed infection with drug-susceptible and drug-resistant TB strains could however, interfere with the accurate phenotypic and/or genotypic diagnosis of TB drug resistance (as highlighted in Chapter 6 and 7 of this book) [60]. Additionally, a more detailed understanding of how HIV co-infection affects the transmission dynamics of drug resistant TB is needed [67, 146, 358].

The strength of this part of the study was to provide an overview of the molecular epidemiology of RR-TB in Khayelitsha during 2013 to 2015. However, the small sample size, especially for RMR-TB over three years, is a limitation; thus, strain diversity defining subspecies within lineages was not included in this part of the study (Chapter eight). Nonetheless, more data is in the process of being captured for further investigation over a longer duration from RR-TB strains in Khayelitsha. Another limitation of this study is partial sampling or culture selection biases, as sequencing data may have not been a true representation of the presence of *M.tb* in the re-cultured MGIT from patient isolates; hence, not representing the overall diversity of the initial sputum sample and within-patient diversity [63, 120] Other sampling difficulties (including those with high bacterial loads) may include human contamination and commensal microbial reads, that could potentially prevent adequate depth coverage of *M.tb* genomes and reliable variant calling [120, 133, 281]. This might have influenced the overall transmission cluster analysis in this part of the study (Chapter eight). To overcome this in future studies, deep sequencing and examination of minor variants could help reveal diversity in the context of transmission. Lastly, the impact of migration on transmission factors in Khayelitsha is, as yet, not understood, as many patients move to and from other areas, specifically the Eastern Cape province in South Africa. More investigation is needed in this regard.

## 9.2 Conclusion

In conclusion, these results either suggest that RMR-TB has a lower tendency to transmit; or that RMR-TB emerged more recently over the years, thus, having less time to develop compensation for fitness loss and consequent increased transmissibility; than for MDR-TB in Khayelitsha during 2013 to 2015. Despite the limited sample size, RMR-TB has shown 50% transmission among the disputed *rpoB* L511P mutation, with low-level rifampicin resistance; rarely reported in other settings. This raises concern, as *rpoB* L511P was found to be one of the most predominant strains circulating among RMR-TB patients in Khayelitsha during 2013 to 2015; as this disputed mutation is often not detected by phenotypic drug susceptibility testing. Hence, this may cause significant implications for the treatment and clinical care of RR-TB patients (as discussed in Chapter 7). Furthermore, there is limited data on the transmission of RMR-TB, especially in African countries (as highlighted in the systematic review, Chapter 4).

Additionally, among all RR-TB we found that MDR-TB; specifically among *rpoB* S531L (Lineage2); is highly transmissible in Khayelitsha; also, commonly found in many other settings [343, 344, 353]. Cox *et al.* [43] suggest that HIV in high TB prevalence settings (such as Khayelitsha) is driving both drug-susceptible and drug-resistant TB transmission. However, in order to assist in the reduction of transmission of drug resistant TB, the following has been suggested – early identification and treatment of DR-TB patients, education and awareness about DR-TB transmission to household members, screening of household contacts, and good infection control practises in congregate settings [359]. Other issues that still need to be addressed are proper treatment regimens (ideally individualized TB treatment for patients); including implementation of WGS in routinely diagnosed low-income, high incident DR-TB settings; and improved accessibility for patients to provide better treatment outcomes, especially among HIV positive individuals.

# CHAPTER TEN

## 10. Key findings and general conclusions

Since South Africa shows high and increasing prevalence of RMR-TB (Chapter one: Introduction), this doctoral research study aimed to describe RMR-TB in more detail within Khayelitsha, a peri-urban township in Cape Town, the Western Cape Province, South Africa. Within this book, the systematic review (Chapter four: section on temporal trends) highlights that RMR-TB varies significantly across different settings and constitutes a large proportion of the rifampicin-resistant TB (RR-TB) burden globally. Within the nine provinces of South Africa, considerable variation in the increase of rifampicin mono-resistant TB (RMR-TB) over time, among either RR-TB, or all TB was found (Chapter four: section on temporal trends). Although studies were limited on RMR-TB in the systematic review of this book, findings showed that most of the data from high HIV prevalence settings came from South Africa.

By analysing clinical data over a decade, chapter five of this book (Epidemiology of RMR-TB in Khayelitsha), has shown that the prevalence of routinely diagnosed RR-TB (including RMR- and MDR-TB), remained relatively stable with no major temporal trend observed. In chapter five, when assessing clinical data together with additional data received from the Provincial Health Data Centre (PHDC) Western Cape over a three-year cohort, findings suggest that there may be a higher risk of rifampicin resistance (RIF R) acquisition during first-line TB treatment among HIV positive individuals compared to those who are HIV negative. Similarly, studies from the systematic review (Chapter four: section on risk factors) found that HIV positivity was significantly associated with RMR-TB among both RR-TB and all TB, regardless of whether individuals had a previous TB treatment history or not.

In the sixth and seventh chapter of this book (Mutations in *rpoB* and MICs among RR-TB strains), a high proportion of discordance between genotypic and phenotypic testing, resulting from possible mixed infections and/or false-positive RIF R diagnosis was found. Although the impact of mixed infections on treatment outcomes remains unclear, this may potentially lead to poorer treatment outcomes among RR-TB patients, as there is often a delay in the treatment process among these patients due to laboratory discordances found, with the additional difficulty from the clinician in making decisions in treating these patients, without the possibility of overtreating patients with false-positive RR-TB. This part of the study also found that the DR-TB profile (based on whole genome sequencing - WGS) for *rpoB* mutations were distinctly different between RMR- and MDR-TB strains. Hence, this suggests a difference in the evolutionary mechanism of RIF R between RMR- and MDR-TB strains; and could result in different treatment approaches and clinical care between RMR- and MDR-TB patients. Furthermore, the proportion of high/moderate versus minimal confidence levels for *rpoB* mutations was significantly higher among MDR-TB; specifically, high confidence mutation *rpoB* S531L (Lineage 2); than for RMR-TB. This part of the study also found that among RMR-TB strains, *rpoB* L511P (described as a disputed mutation, conferring minimal confidence for RIF R or low-level RIF R) was more prevalent among RMR-TB than for MDR-TB. All *rpoB* L511P mutations (including RMR- and MDR-TB) tested phenotypically susceptible to rifampicin with the mycobacteria growth indicator tube (MGIT) quantitative phenotypic DST (q pDST); causing discrepancies between WGS and q pDST. Lastly, all RMR-TB strains, including those with *rpoB* L511P mutations, had no other mutations conferring resistance to any of the other TB drugs. Thus, this too could result in significant implications for the treatment and clinical care of RR-TB patients.

When conducting the systematic review (Chapter four: section on transmission), it was evident that studies on RMR-TB transmission are limited. Hence, studies from this section of the systematic review clearly illustrate that RMR-TB transmission occurs in both high and low HIV prevalence countries, and that RMR-TB may have a lower tendency to transmit than for MDR-TB. Despite the limited sample size of only three years of data for performing transmission cluster analysis in the study cohort (Chapter eight and nine), it is apparent that RMR-TB may be less transmissible than MDR-TB as initially hypothesized in this book. More MDR-TB strains clustered among *rpoB* S531L (high confidence mutation) compared to RMR-TB with the same mutation. In contrast, among *rpoB* L511P (minimal/low confidence mutation) more RMR-TB strains clustered compared to no clustering found among MDR-TB strains with the same mutation. Clinical information showed that RMR-TB *rpoB* L511P clusters were either due to closely related community acquired or nosocomial transmission, with no evidence of household contacts in any of the clusters. SNP differences were also less than five, suggesting direct transmission between RMR-TB patients where the *rpoB* L511P mutation is present. Hence, it is evident that in the setting of Khayelitsha, low-level disputed *rpoB* L511P mutations are transmitting to some degree, which also causes concern for the treatment and clinical care of RR-TB patients.

Based on these key findings, future studies could include investigating the optimisation of RR-TB treatment for patients with RMR-TB, especially among HIV and TB co-infected patients, and patients with low-level RIF R or disputed *rpoB* mutations. Currently higher doses of rifampicin or substitution with rifabutin has been suggested for treatment of these patients but has not been further investigated in terms of clinical outcomes. Patient centred care could also help to improve patient treatment outcomes as optimal drug regimens, especially for low-level and discordant RR-TB are currently undefined.

Even though WGS is currently not routinely available in resource-limited settings such as South Africa, it could be beneficial to be used in conjunction with minimum inhibitory concentration (MIC) testing for individualised patient treatment regimens, in order to accurately diagnosis RR-TB in the near future. This book also highlights the importance of future work such as direct WGS of *M.tb* isolated directly from specimens, which may assist in determining low-level RIF R, heteroresistance and/or false-positive RIF R, with an added benefit of identifying single nucleotide variants (SNVs) (to detect silent mutations), for better diagnosis of RIF R. An additional benefit of WGS in this instance would be to better understand transmission among RR-TB, especially among RMR-TB patients. In general, the key to preventing *M.tb* (drug-susceptible and drug-resistant) transmission; irrespective of HIV status; is rapid diagnosis and treatment initiation, together with the development and implementation of infection control programmes to reduce nosocomial, household and community acquired transmission.

In conclusion, this book presents an understanding of RR-TB strains (specifically RMR- and MDR-TB) during 2013 to 2015 in Khayelitsha. The findings presented in this book add new insights in the setting of Khayelitsha, that could assist in improving case detection and treatment outcomes, by providing knowledge of the acquisition and transmission of RIF R, as well as deciphering possible discordance such as mixed infections between genotypic and phenotypic testing. To better understand the implications of the results presented in this book, future work from the broader Khayelitsha study will include performing research on the knowledge gaps concluded from this research study; by investigating a much larger subset of strains. Thus, it would be beneficial to gain a better perspective over a larger time period within Khayelitsha.

Prospective research gathered from the findings of this book may include:

- Further investigation on the impact of HIV on rifampicin resistance acquisition; including other possible risk factors found; among RR-TB (RMR- and MDR-TB) patients.
- Further research on whether presumed cases of acquired rifampicin-resistance acquisition correlate with WGS transmission cluster analysis among RR-TB patients over a long time period is required.
- Determining the distribution of *rpoB* mutations among RR-TB (RMR- and MDR-TB); including detection of any compensatory mutations and their association with transmission.

- Further research performed on MICs (with comparison of liquid MGIT and solid agar proportion methods) among *rpoB* L511P and other disputed mutations, to further investigate low-level RIF R and discordance between genotypic and phenotypic testing.
- Further investigation of mixed infections or heterogeneity among RR-TB isolates with significant discordance between WGS-based DST and routine DST.
- Investigating different pathways to the emergence of RMR-TB in comparison to MDR-TB, and the relative transmission of these RR-TB strains.

# References


1. Organization, W.H., *Definitions and reporting framework for tuberculosis–2013 revision*. 2013, World Health Organization.
2. WHO, *Global Tuberculosis report 2019; World Health Organization, Geneva.*
3. WHO, *Global Tuberculosis report 2016; World Health Organization, Geneva.*
4. Ismail, N.A., et al., *Prevalence of drug-resistant tuberculosis and imputed burden in South Africa: a national and sub-national cross-sectional survey.* The Lancet Infectious Diseases, 2018. **18**(7): p. 779-787.
5. Diseases, N.I.f.C., *South African tuberculosis drug resistance survey 2012-14*. 2016, National Institute for Communicable Diseases Johannesburg.
6. Katende, B., et al., *Rifampicin Resistant tuberculosis in Lesotho: Diagnosis, treatment initiation and outcomes.* Scientific Reports, 2020. **10**(1): p. 1-8.
7. Mvelase, N.R., et al., *Evolving rifampicin and isoniazid mono-resistance in a high multidrug-resistant and extensively drug-resistant tuberculosis region: a retrospective data analysis.* BMJ open, 2019. **9**(11).
8. Kendall, E.A., M.O. Fofana, and D.W. Dowdy, *Burden of transmitted multidrug resistance in epidemics of tuberculosis: a transmission modelling analysis.* Lancet Respir Med, 2015. **3**(12): p. 963-72.
9. Borrell, S. and S. Gagneux, *Infectiousness, reproductive fitness and evolution of drug-resistant Mycobacterium tuberculosis [State of the art].* The International Journal of Tuberculosis and Lung Disease, 2009. **13**(12): p. 1456-1466.
10. Suen, S.-c., E. Bendavid, and J.D. Goldhaber-Fiebert, *Disease Control Implications of India's Changing Multi-Drug Resistant Tuberculosis Epidemic.* Plos One, 2014. **9**(3).
11. Andersson, D.I. and B.R. Levin, *The biological cost of antibiotic resistance.* Curr Opin Microbiol, 1999. **2**(5): p. 489-93.
12. David, H.L., *Probability distribution of drug-resistant mutants in unselected populations of Mycobacterium tuberculosis.* Appl. Environ. Microbiol., 1970. **20**(5): p. 810-814.
13. Andersson, D.I. and D. Hughes, *Antibiotic resistance and its cost: is it possible to reverse resistance?* Nature Reviews Microbiology, 2010. **8**(4): p. 260-271.
14. Böttger, E.C. and B. Springer, *Tuberculosis: drug resistance, fitness, and strategies for global control.* European journal of pediatrics, 2008. **167**(2): p. 141-148.
15. Dye, C., et al., *Erasing the world's slow stain: strategies to beat multidrug-resistant tuberculosis.* Science, 2002. **295**(5562): p. 2042-2046.
16. Cohen, T., B. Sommers, and M. Murray, *The effect of drug resistance on the fitness of Mycobacterium tuberculosis.* The Lancet infectious diseases, 2003. **3**(1): p. 13-21.
17. Borrell, S. and S. Gagneux, *Strain diversity, epistasis and the evolution of drug resistance in Mycobacterium tuberculosis.* Clinical Microbiology and Infection, 2011. **17**(6): p. 815-820.
18. Ramaswamy, S. and J.M. Musser, *Molecular genetic basis of antimicrobial agent resistance inMycobacterium tuberculosis: 1998 update.* Tubercle and Lung Disease, 1998. **79**(1): p. 3-29.
19. Somoskovi, A., L.M. Parsons, and M. Salfinger, *The molecular basis of resistance to isoniazid, rifampin, and pyrazinamide in Mycobacterium tuberculosis.* Respiratory research, 2001. **2**(3): p. 164.
20. Telenti, A., et al., *Detection of rifampicin-resistance mutations in Mycobacterium tuberculosis.* The Lancet, 1993. **341**(8846): p. 647-651.
21. Ezekiel, D.H. and J.E. Hutchins, *Mutations affecting RNA polymerase associated with rifampicin resistance in Escherichia coli.* Nature, 1968. **220**(5164): p. 276-277.
22. Pierre-Audigier, C. and B. Gicquel, *The contribution of molecular biology in diagnosing tuberculosis and detecting antibiotic resistance.* 2012.

23. André, E., et al., *Consensus numbering system for the rifampicin resistance-associated rpoB gene mutations in pathogenic mycobacteria.* Clinical Microbiology and Infection, 2017. **23**(3): p. 167-172.
24. Van Deun, A., et al., *Mycobacterium tuberculosis strains with highly discordant rifampin susceptibility test results.* Journal of clinical microbiology, 2009. **47**(11): p. 3501-3506.
25. Pang, Y., et al., *Study of the rifampin monoresistance mechanism in Mycobacterium tuberculosis.* Antimicrobial agents and chemotherapy, 2013. **57**(2): p. 893-900.
26. Rigouts, L., et al., *Rifampin resistance missed in automated liquid culture system for Mycobacterium tuberculosis isolates with specific rpoB mutations.* J Clin Microbiol, 2013. **51**(8): p. 2641-5.
27. Van Deun, A., et al., *Disputed rpoB mutations can frequently cause important rifampicin resistance among new tuberculosis patients.* The International Journal of Tuberculosis and Lung Disease, 2015. **19**(2): p. 185-190.
28. Jamieson, F.B., et al., *Profiling of Mutations and MICs for Rifampin and Rifabutin in Mycobacterium tuberculosis.* Journal of Clinical Microbiology, 2014. **52**(6): p. 2157-2162.
29. Heep, M., et al., *Frequency of rpoB Mutations Inside and Outside the Cluster I Region in Rifampin-Resistant Clinical Mycobacterium tuberculosis Isolates.* Journal of Clinical Microbiology, 2001. **39**(1): p. 107-110.
30. Sanchez-Padilla, E., et al., *Detection of Drug-Resistant Tuberculosis by Xpert MTB/RIF in Swaziland.* New England Journal of Medicine, 2015. **372**(12): p. 1181-1182.
31. Van Deun, A., et al., *Rifampin drug resistance tests for tuberculosis: challenging the gold standard.* J Clin Microbiol, 2013. **51**(8): p. 2633-40.
32. Zignol, M., et al., *Genetic sequencing for surveillance of drug resistance in tuberculosis in highly endemic countries: a multi-country population-based surveillance study.* The Lancet Infectious Diseases, 2018. **18**(6): p. 675-683.
33. Ahmad, S., N.M. Al-Mutairi, and E. Mokaddas, *Variations in the occurrence of specific rpoB mutations in rifampicin-resistant Mycobacterium tuberculosis isolates from patients of different ethnic groups in Kuwait.* Indian J Med Res, 2012. **135**(5): p. 756-62.
34. *World Health Organisation. Companion handbook to the WHO guidelines for the programmatic management of drug-resistant tuberculosis. Geneva: WHO.* http://www.who.int/tb/publications/pmdt_companionhandbook/en/, 2014.
35. Shah, N.S., et al., *Transmission of extensively drug-resistant tuberculosis in South Africa.* New England Journal of Medicine, 2017. **376**(3): p. 243-253.
36. Bhembe, N.L. and E. Green, *Molecular epidemiological study of multidrug-resistant tuberculosis isolated from sputum samples in Eastern Cape, South Africa.* Infection, Genetics and Evolution, 2020: p. 104182.
37. Rockwood, N., et al., *Risk factors for acquired rifamycin and isoniazid resistance: a systematic review and meta-analysis.* PLoS One, 2015. **10**(9).
38. Gandhi, N.R., et al., *Multidrug-resistant and extensively drug-resistant tuberculosis: a threat to global control of tuberculosis.* The Lancet, 2010. **375**(9728): p. 1830-1843.
39. Pillay, M. and A.W. Sturm, *Evolution of the extensively drug-resistant F15/LAM4/KZN strain of Mycobacterium tuberculosis in KwaZulu-Natal, South Africa.* Clinical infectious diseases, 2007. **45**(11): p. 1409-1414.
40. Calver, A.D., et al., *Emergence of increased resistance and extensively drug-resistant tuberculosis despite treatment adherence, South Africa.* Emerging infectious diseases, 2010. **16**(2): p. 264.
41. Klopper, M., et al., *Emergence and spread of extensively and totally drug-resistant tuberculosis, South Africa.* Emerging infectious diseases, 2013. **19**(3): p. 449.
42. Van Rie, A., et al., *Classification of drug-resistant tuberculosis in an epidemic area.* The Lancet, 2000. **356**(9223): p. 22-25.

43. Cox, H.S., et al., *Epidemic Levels of Drug Resistant Tuberculosis (MDR and XDR-TB) in a High HIV Prevalence Setting in Khayelitsha, South Africa.* Plos One, 2010. **5**(11).
44. Blomberg, B., et al., *The rationale for recommending fixed-dose combination tablets for treatment of tuberculosis.* Bulletin of the world health organization, 2001. **79**: p. 61-68.
45. Caudron, J.M., et al., *Substandard medicines in resource-poor settings: a problem that can no longer be ignored.* Tropical Medicine & International Health, 2008. **13**(8): p. 1062-1072.
46. Laserson, K., et al., *Substandard tuberculosis drugs on the global market and their simple detection.* The International Journal of Tuberculosis and Lung Disease, 2001. **5**(5): p. 448-454.
47. Srivastava, S., et al., *Multidrug-resistant tuberculosis not due to noncompliance but to between-patient pharmacokinetic variability.* J Infect Dis, 2011. **204**(12): p. 1951-9.
48. Lutfey, M., et al., *Independent origin of mono-rifampin-resistant Mycobacterium tuberculosis in patients with AIDS.* Am J Respir Crit Care Med, 1996. **153**(2): p. 837-40.
49. Trapnell, C.B., et al., *Increased plasma rifabutin levels with concomitant fluconazole therapy in HIV-infected patients.* Annals of internal medicine, 1996. **124**(6): p. 573-576.
50. Tappero, J.W., et al., *Serum concentrations of antimycobacterial drugs in patients with pulmonary tuberculosis in Botswana.* Clinical infectious diseases, 2005. **41**(4): p. 461-469.
51. Barnes, P.F., *The Influence of Epidemiologic Factors on Drug Resistance Rates in Tuberculosis1• 2.* Am Rev Respir Dis, 1987. **136**: p. 325-328.
52. Gordin, F.M., et al., *The impact of human immunodeficiency virus infection on drug-resistant tuberculosis.* American journal of respiratory and critical care medicine, 1996. **154**(5): p. 1478-1483.
53. Reichman, L.B., *Tuberculosis elimination--what's to stop us?* The international Journal of Tuberculosis and lung disease, 1997. **1**(1): p. 3-11.
54. De Steenwinkel, J., et al., *Drug susceptibility of Mycobacterium tuberculosis Beijing genotype and association with MDR TB.* 2012.
55. Guerra-Assunção, J.A., et al., *Recurrence due to relapse or reinfection with Mycobacterium tuberculosis: a whole-genome sequencing approach in a large, population-based cohort with a high HIV infection prevalence and active follow-up.* The Journal of infectious diseases, 2015. **211**(7): p. 1154-1163.
56. Lambert, M.-L., et al., *Recurrence in tuberculosis: relapse or reinfection?* The Lancet infectious diseases, 2003. **3**(5): p. 282-287.
57. Schiroli, C., et al., *Exogenous reinfection of tuberculosis in a low-burden area.* Infection, 2015. **43**(6): p. 647-653.
58. Small, P.M., et al., *Exogenous reinfection with multidrug-resistant Mycobacterium tuberculosis in patients with advanced HIV infection.* New England Journal of Medicine, 1993. **328**(16): p. 1137-1144.
59. van Rie, A., et al., *Reinfection and mixed infection cause changing Mycobacterium tuberculosis drug-resistance patterns.* American journal of respiratory and critical care medicine, 2005. **172**(5): p. 636-642.
60. Metcalfe, J.Z., et al., *Cryptic microheteroresistance explains Mycobacterium tuberculosis phenotypic resistance.* American journal of respiratory and critical care medicine, 2017. **196**(9): p. 1191-1201.
61. Cohen, T., et al., *Within-host heterogeneity of Mycobacterium tuberculosis infection is associated with poor early treatment response: a prospective cohort study.* The Journal of infectious diseases, 2016. **213**(11): p. 1796-1799.
62. Hanekom, M., et al., *Population structure of mixed Mycobacterium tuberculosis infection is strain genotype and culture medium dependent.* PLoS one, 2013. **8**(7): p. e70178.
63. Hatherell, H.-A., et al., *Interpreting whole genome sequencing for investigating tuberculosis transmission: a systematic review.* BMC medicine, 2016. **14**: p. 21-21.

64. Zhao, M., et al., *Transmission of MDR and XDR tuberculosis in Shanghai, China.* PloS one, 2009. **4**(2).
65. Mariam, D.H., et al., *Effect of rpoB Mutations Conferring Rifampin Resistance on Fitness of Mycobacterium tuberculosis.* Antimicrobial Agents and Chemotherapy, 2004. **48**(4): p. 1289-1294.
66. de Lourdes García-García, M., et al., *Clinical consequences and transmissibility of drug-resistant tuberculosis in southern Mexico.* Archives of internal medicine, 2000. **160**(5): p. 630-636.
67. Khan, P.Y., et al., *Transmission of drug-resistant tuberculosis in HIV-endemic settings.* The Lancet Infectious Diseases, 2019. **19**(3): p. e77-e88.
68. Dadu, A., et al., *Drug-resistant tuberculosis in eastern Europe and central Asia: a time-series analysis of routine surveillance data.* The Lancet Infectious Diseases, 2020. **20**(2): p. 250-258.
69. Yang, C., et al., *Transmission of multidrug-resistant Mycobacterium tuberculosis in Shanghai, China: a retrospective observational study using whole-genome sequencing and epidemiological investigation.* The Lancet Infectious Diseases, 2017. **17**(3): p. 275-284.
70. Merker, M., et al., *Compensatory evolution drives multidrug-resistant tuberculosis in Central Asia.* Elife, 2018. **7**: p. e38200.
71. Frieden, T.R., et al., *A multi-institutional outbreak of highly drug-resistant tuberculosis: epidemiology and clinical outcomes.* Jama, 1996. **276**(15): p. 1229-1235.
72. Gandhi, N.R., et al., *Nosocomial transmission of extensively drug-resistant tuberculosis in a rural hospital in South Africa.* The Journal of infectious diseases, 2013. **207**(1): p. 9-17.
73. Vella, V., et al., *Household contact investigation of multidrug-resistant and extensively drug-resistant tuberculosis in a high HIV prevalence setting.* The International journal of tuberculosis and lung disease, 2011. **15**(9): p. 1170-1175.
74. Teixeira, L., et al., *Infection and disease among household contacts of patients with multidrug-resistant tuberculosis.* The International Journal of Tuberculosis and Lung Disease, 2001. **5**(4): p. 321-328.
75. Grandjean, L., et al., *Transmission of multidrug-resistant and drug-susceptible tuberculosis within households: a prospective cohort study.* PLoS medicine, 2015. **12**(6).
76. Dheda, K., et al., *The epidemiology, pathogenesis, transmission, diagnosis, and management of multidrug-resistant, extensively drug-resistant, and incurable tuberculosis.* The lancet Respiratory medicine, 2017. **5**(4): p. 291-360.
77. Gardy, J.L., et al., *Whole-genome sequencing and social-network analysis of a tuberculosis outbreak.* New England Journal of Medicine, 2011. **364**(8): p. 730-739.
78. Andrews, J.R., et al., *Integrating social contact and environmental data in evaluating tuberculosis transmission in a South African township.* The Journal of infectious diseases, 2014. **210**(4): p. 597-603.
79. Robertson, S., et al., *Tuberculosis in a South African prison–a transmission modelling analysis.* South African Medical Journal, 2011. **101**(11): p. 809-813.
80. Basu, S., et al., *The production of consumption: addressing the impact of mineral mining on tuberculosis in southern Africa.* Globalization and health, 2009. **5**(1): p. 11.
81. Shah, I., V. Poojari, and H. Meshram, *Multi-Drug Resistant and Extensively-Drug Resistant Tuberculosis.* The Indian Journal of Pediatrics, 2020: p. 1-7.
82. Demers, A.-M., et al., *Direct susceptibility testing of Mycobacterium tuberculosis for pyrazinamide by use of the bactec MGIT 960 system.* Journal of clinical microbiology, 2016. **54**(5): p. 1276-1281.
83. Organization, W.H., *The use of next-generation sequencing technologies for the detection of mutations associated with drug resistance in Mycobacterium tuberculosis complex: technical guide.* 2018, World Health Organization.

84. Morgan, M., et al., *A commercial line probe assay for the rapid detection of rifampicin resistance in Mycobacterium tuberculosis: a systematic review and meta-analysis.* BMC infectious diseases, 2005. **5**(1): p. 62.
85. Steingart, K.R., et al., *Xpert® MTB/RIF assay for pulmonary tuberculosis and rifampicin resistance in adults.* Cochrane database of systematic reviews, 2013(1).
86. SADOH, *Interim clinical guidance for the implementation of injectablefree regimens for rifampicin-resistant tubercuosis in adults, adolescents and children.* . South African Department of Health., 2018. http://www.tbonline.info/media/uploads/documents/dr_tb_clinical_guidelines_for_rsa_september_2018.pdf.
87. Van Rie, A., et al., *Discordances between molecular assays for rifampicin resistance in Mycobacterium tuberculosis: frequency, mechanisms and clinical impact.* Journal of Antimicrobial Chemotherapy, 2020. **75**(5): p. 1123-1129.
88. Hanrahan, C.F., et al., *The impact of expanded testing for multidrug resistant tuberculosis using genotype [correction of geontype] MTBDRplus in South Africa: an observational cohort study.* PLoS One, 2012. **7**(11): p. e49898.
89. Coovadia, Y.M., et al., *Rifampicin mono-resistance in Mycobacterium tuberculosis in KwaZulu-Natal, South Africa: a significant phenomenon in a high prevalence TB-HIV region.* PLoS One, 2013. **8**(11): p. e77712.
90. Kendall, E.A., et al., *Estimated clinical impact of the Xpert MTB/RIF Ultra cartridge for diagnosis of pulmonary tuberculosis: a modeling study.* PLoS medicine, 2017. **14**(12): p. e1002472.
91. Zhou, C., et al., *Factors that determine catastrophic expenditure for tuberculosis care: a patient survey in China.* Infectious diseases of poverty, 2016. **5**(1): p. 1-10.
92. Moreira, J., et al., *Weighing harm in therapeutic decisions of smear-negative pulmonary tuberculosis.* Medical Decision Making, 2009. **29**(3): p. 380-390.
93. Pinto, L. and D. Menzies, *Treatment of drug-resistant tuberculosis.* Infection and drug resistance, 2011. **4**: p. 129.
94. Richter, E., S. Rüsch-Gerdes, and D. Hillemann, *Drug-susceptibility testing in TB: current status and future prospects.* Expert Review of Respiratory Medicine, 2009. **3**(5): p. 497-510.
95. Cambau, E., et al., *Revisiting susceptibility testing in MDR-TB by a standardized quantitative phenotypic assessment in a European multicentre study.* Journal of Antimicrobial Chemotherapy, 2015. **70**(3): p. 686-696.
96. Böttger, E., *The ins and outs of Mycobacterium tuberculosis drug susceptibility testing.* Clinical microbiology and infection, 2011. **17**(8): p. 1128-1134.
97. Ängeby, K., et al., *Challenging a dogma: antimicrobial susceptibility testing breakpoints for Mycobacterium tuberculosis.* Bulletin of the World Health Organization, 2012. **90**: p. 693-698.
98. Canetti, G., et al., *Mycobacteria: laboratory methods for testing drug sensitivity and resistance.* Bulletin of the World Health Organization, 1963. **29**(5): p. 565.
99. Canetti, G., et al., *Advances in techniques of testing mycobacterial drug sensitivity, and the use of sensitivity tests in tuberculosis control programmes.* Bulletin of the World Health Organization, 1969. **41**(1): p. 21.
100. Siddiqi, S. and S. Rusch-Gerdes, *MGIT procedure manual for BACTEC MGIT 960 TB system (also applicable for manual MGIT).* Becton, Dickinson, Franklin Lakes, NJ, 2006.
101. Springer Burkhard , L.K., Calligaris-Maibach Romana ,Ritter Claudia ,C. Böttger Erik *Quantitative Drug Susceptibility Testing of Mycobacterium tuberculosis by Use of MGIT 960 and EpiCenter Instrumentation.* J Clin Microbiol, 2009. **Jun; 47(6):** : p. 1773–1780.
102. Miotto, P., D.M. Cirillo, and G.B. Migliori, *Drug resistance in Mycobacterium tuberculosis: molecular mechanisms challenging fluoroquinolones and pyrazinamide effectiveness.* Chest, 2015. **147**(4): p. 1135-1143.

103. Stavrum, R., et al., *High diversity of Mycobacterium tuberculosis genotypes in South Africa and preponderance of mixed infections among ST53 isolates.* Journal of clinical microbiology, 2009. **47**(6): p. 1848-1856.
104. Van Embden, J., et al., *Strain identification of Mycobacterium tuberculosis by DNA fingerprinting: recommendations for a standardized methodology.* Journal of clinical microbiology, 1993. **31**(2): p. 406-409.
105. Small, P.M., et al., *The Epidemiology of Tuberculosis in San Francisco--A Population-Based Study Using Conventional and Molecular Methods.* New England Journal of Medicine, 1994. **330**(24): p. 1703-1709.
106. Alland, D., et al., *Transmission of tuberculosis in New York City--an analysis by DNA fingerprinting and conventional epidemiologic methods.* New England Journal of Medicine, 1994. **330**(24): p. 1710-1716.
107. Van der Spuy, G. and R. Warren, *Molecular epidemiology of Mycobacterium tuberculosis.* Analysis and application of evolutionary markers in the epidemiology of Mycobacterium tuberculosis, 2008: p. 1.
108. Brudey, K., et al., *Mycobacterium tuberculosis complex genetic diversity: mining the fourth international spoligotyping database (SpolDB4) for classification, population genetics and epidemiology.* BMC microbiology, 2006. **6**(1): p. 23.
109. Barnes, P.F. and M.D. Cave, *Molecular epidemiology of tuberculosis.* New England Journal of Medicine, 2003. **349**(12): p. 1149-1156.
110. Allix, C., P. Supply, and M. Fauville-Dufaux, *Utility of fast mycobacterial interspersed repetitive unit—variable number tandem repeat genotyping in clinical mycobacteriological analysis.* Clinical infectious diseases, 2004. **39**(6): p. 783-789.
111. Mears, J., et al., *The prospective evaluation of the TB strain typing service in England: a mixed methods study.* Thorax, 2016. **71**(8): p. 734-741.
112. Gurjav, U., et al., *Whole genome sequencing demonstrates limited transmission within identified Mycobacterium tuberculosis clusters in New South Wales, Australia.* PloS one, 2016. **11**(10).
113. Hirsh, A.E., et al., *Stable association between strains of Mycobacterium tuberculosis and their human host populations.* Proceedings of the National Academy of Sciences, 2004. **101**(14): p. 4871-4876.
114. Mostowy, S., et al., *Genomic analysis distinguishes Mycobacterium africanum.* Journal of clinical microbiology, 2004. **42**(8): p. 3594-3599.
115. Mostowy, S., D. Cousins, and M.A. Behr, *Genomic interrogation of the dassie bacillus reveals it as a unique RD1 mutant within the Mycobacterium tuberculosis complex.* Journal of bacteriology, 2004. **186**(1): p. 104-109.
116. Tsolaki, A.G., et al., *Functional and evolutionary genomics of Mycobacterium tuberculosis: insights from genomic deletions in 100 strains.* Proceedings of the National Academy of Sciences, 2004. **101**(14): p. 4865-4870.
117. Gagneux, S., et al., *Variable host–pathogen compatibility in Mycobacterium tuberculosis.* Proceedings of the National Academy of Sciences, 2006. **103**(8): p. 2869-2873.
118. Tsolaki, A.G., et al., *Genomic deletions classify the Beijing/W strains as a distinct genetic lineage of Mycobacterium tuberculosis.* Journal of clinical microbiology, 2005. **43**(7): p. 3185-3191.
119. Alland, D., et al., *Role of large sequence polymorphisms (LSPs) in generating genomic diversity among clinical isolates of Mycobacterium tuberculosis and the utility of LSPs in phylogenetic analysis.* Journal of clinical microbiology, 2007. **45**(1): p. 39-46.
120. Meehan, C.J., et al., *Whole genome sequencing of Mycobacterium tuberculosis: current standards and open issues.* Nature Reviews Microbiology, 2019. **17**(9): p. 533-545.

121. Dolinger, D.L., et al., *Next-generation sequencing-based user-friendly platforms for drug-resistant tuberculosis diagnosis: a promise for the near future.* International journal of mycobacteriology, 2016. **5**: p. S27-S28.
122. Farhat, M.R., et al., *Genomic analysis identifies targets of convergent positive selection in drug-resistant Mycobacterium tuberculosis.* Nat Genet, 2013. **45**(10): p. 1183-9.
123. Lanzas, F., et al., *Multidrug-resistant tuberculosis in panama is driven by clonal expansion of a multidrug-resistant Mycobacterium tuberculosis strain related to the KZN extensively drug-resistant M. tuberculosis strain from South Africa.* J Clin Microbiol, 2013. **51**(10): p. 3277-85.
124. Casali, N., et al., *Evolution and transmission of drug-resistant tuberculosis in a Russian population.* Nat Genet, 2014. **46**(3): p. 279-86.
125. Casali, N., et al., *Microevolution of extensively drug-resistant tuberculosis in Russia.* Genome Res, 2012. **22**(4): p. 735-45.
126. Zhang, H., et al., *Genome sequencing of 161 Mycobacterium tuberculosis isolates from China identifies genes and intergenic regions associated with drug resistance.* Nat Genet, 2013. **45**(10): p. 1255-60.
127. Niemann, S. and P. Supply, *Diversity and evolution of Mycobacterium tuberculosis: moving to whole-genome-based approaches.* Cold Spring Harbor perspectives in medicine, 2014. **4**(12): p. a021188.
128. Walker, T.M., et al., *Whole-genome sequencing for prediction of Mycobacterium tuberculosis drug susceptibility and resistance: a retrospective cohort study.* The Lancet infectious diseases, 2015. **15**(10): p. 1193-1202.
129. Köser, C.U., et al., *Routine use of microbial whole genome sequencing in diagnostic and public health microbiology.* PLoS pathogens, 2012. **8**(8).
130. Revez, J., et al., *Survey on the use of whole-genome sequencing for infectious diseases surveillance: rapid expansion of European national capacities, 2015–2016.* Frontiers in public health, 2017. **5**: p. 347.
131. Pankhurst, L.J., et al., *Rapid, comprehensive, and affordable mycobacterial diagnosis with whole-genome sequencing: a prospective study.* The Lancet Respiratory Medicine, 2016. **4**(1): p. 49-58.
132. Votintseva, A.A., et al., *Same-day diagnostic and surveillance data for tuberculosis via whole-genome sequencing of direct respiratory samples.* Journal of clinical microbiology, 2017. **55**(5): p. 1285-1298.
133. Doughty, E.L., et al., *Culture-independent detection and characterisation of Mycobacterium tuberculosis and M. africanum in sputum samples using shotgun metagenomics on a benchtop sequencer.* PeerJ, 2014. **2**: p. e585.
134. Brown, A.C., et al., *Rapid whole-genome sequencing of Mycobacterium tuberculosis isolates directly from clinical samples.* Journal of clinical microbiology, 2015. **53**(7): p. 2230-2237.
135. McNerney, R., et al., *Removing the bottleneck in whole genome sequencing of Mycobacterium tuberculosis for rapid drug resistance analysis: a call to action.* International Journal of Infectious Diseases, 2017. **56**: p. 130-135.
136. Walker, T.M., et al., *A cluster of multidrug-resistant Mycobacterium tuberculosis among patients arriving in Europe from the Horn of Africa: a molecular epidemiological study.* Lancet Infect Dis, 2018. **18**(4): p. 431-440.
137. Feuerriegel, S., et al., *PhyResSE: a web tool delineating Mycobacterium tuberculosis antibiotic resistance and lineage from whole-genome sequencing data.* Journal of clinical microbiology, 2015. **53**(6): p. 1908-1914.
138. Steiner, A., et al., *KvarQ: targeted and direct variant calling from fastq reads of bacterial genomes.* BMC genomics, 2014. **15**(1): p. 881.
139. Iwai, H., et al., *CASTB (the comprehensive analysis server for the Mycobacterium tuberculosis complex): A publicly accessible web server for epidemiological analyses, drug-resistance

*prediction and phylogenetic comparison of clinical isolates.* Tuberculosis (Edinburgh, Scotland), 2015. **95**(6): p. 843-844.
140. Mahé, P., et al., *A large scale evaluation of TBProfiler and Mykrobe for antibiotic resistance prediction in Mycobacterium tuberculosis.* PeerJ, 2019. **7**: p. e6857.
141. Phelan, J.E., et al., *Integrating informatics tools and portable sequencing technology for rapid detection of resistance to anti-tuberculous drugs.* Genome medicine, 2019. **11**(1): p. 41-41.
142. Coll, F., et al., *Rapid determination of anti-tuberculosis drug resistance from whole-genome sequences.* Genome medicine, 2015. **7**(1): p. 51.
143. Macedo, R., et al., *Dissecting whole-genome sequencing-based online tools for predicting resistance in Mycobacterium tuberculosis: can we use them for clinical decision guidance?* Tuberculosis, 2018. **110**: p. 44-51.
144. Consortium, C. and G.P. the 100, *Prediction of susceptibility to first-line tuberculosis drugs by DNA sequencing.* New England Journal of Medicine, 2018. **379**(15): p. 1403-1415.
145. Cox, H. and V. Mizrahi, *The coming of age of drug-susceptibility testing for tuberculosis.* 2018, Mass Medical Soc.
146. Walker, T., et al., *Whole genome sequencing for M/XDR tuberculosis surveillance and for resistance testing.* Clinical Microbiology and Infection, 2017. **23**(3): p. 161-166.
147. Miotto, P., et al., *A standardised method for interpreting the association between mutations and phenotypic drug resistance in Mycobacterium tuberculosis.* European Respiratory Journal, 2017. **50**(6): p. 1701354.
148. Hayden, S.R. and M.D. Brown, *Likelihood ratio: a powerful tool for incorporating the results of a diagnostic test into clinical decisionmaking.* Annals of emergency medicine, 1999. **33**(5): p. 575-580.
149. Goodman, S.N., *Toward evidence-based medical statistics. 2: The Bayes factor.* Annals of internal medicine, 1999. **130**(12): p. 1005-1013.
150. Brown, M. and M. Reeves, *Evidence-based emergency medicine/skills for evidence-based emergency care. Interval likelihood ratios: another advantage for the evidence-based diagnostician.* Annals of emergency medicine, 2003. **42**(2): p. 292-297.
151. Guerra-Assunção, J., et al., *Large-scale whole genome sequencing of M. tuberculosis provides insights into transmission in a high prevalence area.* Elife, 2015. **4**: p. e05166.
152. Wollenberg, K.R., et al., *Whole-Genome Sequencing of Mycobacterium tuberculosis Provides Insight into the Evolution and Genetic Composition of Drug-Resistant Tuberculosis in Belarus.* Journal of Clinical Microbiology, 2017. **55**(2): p. 457-469.
153. Senghore, M., et al., *Whole-genome sequencing illuminates the evolution and spread of multidrug-resistant tuberculosis in Southwest Nigeria.* Plos One, 2017. **12**(9).
154. Luo, T., et al., *Whole-genome sequencing to detect recent transmission of Mycobacterium tuberculosis in settings with a high burden of tuberculosis.* Tuberculosis, 2014. **94**(4): p. 434-440.
155. Koch, A., H. Cox, and V. Mizrahi, *Drug-resistant tuberculosis: challenges and opportunities for diagnosis and treatment.* Current opinion in pharmacology, 2018. **42**: p. 7-15.
156. Walker, T.M., et al., *Whole-genome sequencing to delineate Mycobacterium tuberculosis outbreaks: a retrospective observational study.* Lancet Infect Dis, 2013. **13**(2): p. 137-46.
157. Norheim, G., et al., *Tuberculosis outbreak in an educational institution in Norway.* Journal of clinical microbiology, 2017. **55**(5): p. 1327-1333.
158. Bryant, J.M., et al., *Inferring patient to patient transmission of Mycobacterium tuberculosis from whole genome sequencing data.* BMC infectious diseases, 2013. **13**(1): p. 110.
159. Casali, N., et al., *Whole Genome Sequence Analysis of a Large Isoniazid-Resistant Tuberculosis Outbreak in London: A Retrospective Observational Study.* PLoS Med, 2016. **13**(10): p. e1002137.
160. Ford, C., et al., *Mycobacterium tuberculosis–heterogeneity revealed through whole genome sequencing.* Tuberculosis, 2012. **92**(3): p. 194-201.

161. Ford, C.B., et al., *Use of whole genome sequencing to estimate the mutation rate of Mycobacterium tuberculosis during latent infection.* Nature genetics, 2011. **43**(5): p. 482.
162. Walker, T.M., et al., *Assessment of Mycobacterium tuberculosis transmission in Oxfordshire, UK, 2007-12, with whole pathogen genome sequences: an observational study.* Lancet Respir Med, 2014. **2**(4): p. 285-292.
163. Nikolayevskyy, V., et al., *Whole genome sequencing of Mycobacterium tuberculosis for detection of recent transmission and tracing outbreaks: a systematic review.* Tuberculosis, 2016. **98**: p. 77-85.
164. Brites, D. and S. Gagneux, *The nature and evolution of genomic diversity in the Mycobacterium tuberculosis complex*, in *Strain Variation in the Mycobacterium tuberculosis Complex: Its Role in Biology, Epidemiology and Control*. 2017, Springer. p. 1-26.
165. Canetti, G., *Infection caused by atypical mycobacteria and antituberculous immunity.* Lille medical: journal de la Faculte de medecine et de pharmacie de l'Universite de Lille, 1970. **15**(2): p. 280.
166. Van Soolingen, D., et al., *A novel pathogenic taxon of the Mycobacterium tuberculosis complex, Canetti: characterization of an exceptional isolate from Africa.* International Journal of Systematic and Evolutionary Microbiology, 1997. **47**(4): p. 1236-1245.
167. Supply, P., et al., *Genomic analysis of smooth tubercle bacilli provides insights into ancestry and pathoadaptation of Mycobacterium tuberculosis.* Nature genetics, 2013. **45**(2): p. 172-179.
168. Brosch, R., et al., *A new evolutionary scenario for the Mycobacterium tuberculosis complex.* Proceedings of the national academy of Sciences, 2002. **99**(6): p. 3684-3689.
169. De Jong, B.C., M. Antonio, and S. Gagneux, *Mycobacterium africanum—review of an important cause of human tuberculosis in West Africa.* PLoS neglected tropical diseases, 2010. **4**(9).
170. Ngabonziza, J.C.S., et al., *A sister lineage of the Mycobacterium tuberculosis complex discovered in the African Great Lakes region.* Nature Communications, 2020. **11**(1): p. 1-11.
171. Filliol, I., et al., *Global phylogeny of Mycobacterium tuberculosis based on single nucleotide polymorphism (SNP) analysis: insights into tuberculosis evolution, phylogenetic accuracy of other DNA fingerprinting systems, and recommendations for a minimal standard SNP set.* Journal of bacteriology, 2006. **188**(2): p. 759-772.
172. Baker, L., et al., *Silent nucleotide polymorphisms and a phylogeny for Mycobacterium tuberculosis.* Emerging infectious diseases, 2004. **10**(9): p. 1568.
173. Hershberg, R., et al., *High functional diversity in Mycobacterium tuberculosis driven by genetic drift and human demography.* PLoS biology, 2008. **6**(12).
174. Wirth, T., et al., *Origin, spread and demography of the Mycobacterium tuberculosis complex.* PLoS pathogens, 2008. **4**(9).
175. Reed, M.B., et al., *Major Mycobacterium tuberculosis lineages associate with patient country of origin.* Journal of clinical microbiology, 2009. **47**(4): p. 1119-1128.
176. Kohl, T.A., et al., *Whole-genome-based Mycobacterium tuberculosis surveillance: a standardized, portable, and expandable approach.* Journal of clinical microbiology, 2014. **52**(7): p. 2479-2486.
177. Roetzer, A., et al., *Whole genome sequencing versus traditional genotyping for investigation of a Mycobacterium tuberculosis outbreak: a longitudinal molecular epidemiological study.* PLoS medicine, 2013. **10**(2).
178. Török, M.E., et al., *Rapid whole-genome sequencing for investigation of a suspected tuberculosis outbreak.* Journal of clinical microbiology, 2013. **51**(2): p. 611-614.
179. Kato-Maeda, M., et al., *Use of whole genome sequencing to determine the microevolution of Mycobacterium tuberculosis during an outbreak.* PloS one, 2013. **8**(3).
180. Coscolla, M. and S. Gagneux. *Consequences of genomic diversity in Mycobacterium tuberculosis.* in *Seminars in immunology*. 2014. Elsevier.

181. Gagneux, S., *Ecology and evolution of Mycobacterium tuberculosis.* Nature Reviews Microbiology, 2018. **16**(4): p. 202.
182. Cousins, D., et al., *Tuberculosis in imported hyrax (Procavia capensis) caused by an ususual variant belonging to the Mycobacterium tuberculosis complex.* Veterinary microbiology, 1994. **42**(2-3): p. 135-145.
183. Alexander, K.A., et al., *Novel Mycobacterium tuberculosis complex pathogen, M. mungi.* Emerging infectious diseases, 2010. **16**(8): p. 1296.
184. Coscolla, M., et al., *Novel Mycobacterium tuberculosis complex isolate from a wild chimpanzee.* Emerging infectious diseases, 2013. **19**(6): p. 969.
185. Parsons, S.D., et al., *Novel cause of tuberculosis in meerkats, South Africa.* Emerging infectious diseases, 2013. **19**(12): p. 2004.
186. Comas, I., et al., *Out-of-Africa migration and Neolithic coexpansion of Mycobacterium tuberculosis with modern humans.* Nature genetics, 2013. **45**(10): p. 1176.
187. Mahairas, G.G., et al., *Molecular analysis of genetic differences between Mycobacterium bovis BCG and virulent M. bovis.* Journal of bacteriology, 1996. **178**(5): p. 1274-1282.
188. Pym, A.S., et al., *Loss of RD1 contributed to the attenuation of the live tuberculosis vaccines Mycobacterium bovis BCG and Mycobacterium microti.* Molecular microbiology, 2002. **46**(3): p. 709-717.
189. *Strategic Development Information and GIS Department CoCT City of Cape Town 2011 Census - Khayelitsha Health District.* 2013.
190. Health, W.C.D.o., *Western Cape Antenatal HIV Survey 2010.* 2010.
191. Khayelitsha, M.S.F., *Khayelitsha 2001–2011: 10 years of HIV/TB care at primary health care level.* Activity report, 2011. **10**.
192. Cox, H., et al., *Community-based treatment of drug-resistant tuberculosis in Khayelitsha, South Africa.* The International Journal of Tuberculosis and Lung Disease, 2014. **18**(4): p. 441-448.
193. *Sub-district level data 90 90 90 dashboard; Western Cape Provincial Health Department, City of Cape Town Metropolitan Municipality.* 2019.
194. Frontières, M.S., *Decentralized diagnosis and treatment of drug-resistant tuberculosis in Khayelitsha, South Africa.* Outcomes and successes of the decentralized model of care March, 2015.
195. Hughes, J., et al., *Linezolid for multidrug-resistant tuberculosis in HIV-infected and-uninfected patients.* European Respiratory Journal, 2015. **46**(1): p. 271-274.
196. Ndjeka, N., et al., *Treatment of drug-resistant tuberculosis with bedaquiline in a high HIV prevalence setting: an interim cohort analysis.* The International Journal of Tuberculosis and Lung Disease, 2015. **19**(8): p. 979-985.
197. Boulle, A., et al., *Data Centre Profile: The Provincial Health Data Centre of the Western Cape Province, South Africa.* International Journal of Population Data Science, 2019. **4**(2).
198. Warren, R., et al., *Safe Mycobacterium tuberculosis DNA extraction method that does not compromise integrity.* J Clin Microbiol, 2006. **44**(1): p. 254-6.
199. Zaharia, M., et al., *Faster and more accurate sequence alignment with SNAP.* arXiv preprint arXiv:1111.5572, 2011.
200. Coll, F., et al., *A robust SNP barcode for typing Mycobacterium tuberculosis complex strains.* Nature communications, 2014. **5**: p. 4812.
201. Coll, F., et al., *PolyTB: a genomic variation map for Mycobacterium tuberculosis.* Tuberculosis, 2014. **94**(3): p. 346-354.
202. Ocheretina, O., et al., *Correlation between Genotypic and Phenotypic Testing for Resistance to Rifampin in Mycobacterium tuberculosis Clinical Isolates in Haiti: Investigation of Cases with Discrepant Susceptibility Results.* PLOS ONE, 2014. **9**(3): p. e90569.
203. Cock, P.J., et al., *The Sanger FASTQ file format for sequences with quality scores, and the Solexa/Illumina FASTQ variants.* Nucleic acids research, 2009. **38**(6): p. 1767-1771.

204. Bolger, A.M., M. Lohse, and B. Usadel, *Trimmomatic: a flexible trimmer for Illumina sequence data.* Bioinformatics, 2014. **30**(15): p. 2114-2120.
205. Wingett, S.W. and S. Andrews, *FastQ Screen: A tool for multi-genome mapping and quality control.* F1000Research, 2018. **7**.
206. Li, H. and R. Durbin, *Fast and accurate short read alignment with Burrows–Wheeler transform.* bioinformatics, 2009. **25**(14): p. 1754-1760.
207. Li, H., et al., *The sequence alignment/map format and SAMtools.* Bioinformatics, 2009. **25**(16): p. 2078-2079.
208. Koboldt, D.C., et al., *VarScan: variant detection in massively parallel sequencing of individual and pooled samples.* Bioinformatics, 2009. **25**(17): p. 2283-2285.
209. Danecek, P., et al., *The variant call format and VCFtools.* Bioinformatics, 2011. **27**(15): p. 2156-2158.
210. Xu, Y., et al., *High-resolution mapping of tuberculosis transmission: Whole genome sequencing and phylogenetic modelling of a cohort from Valencia Region, Spain.* PLOS Medicine, 2019. **16**(10): p. e1002961.
211. Wang, K., M. Li, and H. Hakonarson, *ANNOVAR: functional annotation of genetic variants from high-throughput sequencing data.* Nucleic acids research, 2010. **38**(16): p. e164-e164.
212. Stamatakis, A., *RAxML version 8: a tool for phylogenetic analysis and post-analysis of large phylogenies.* Bioinformatics, 2014. **30**(9): p. 1312-1313.
213. Rambaut, A., *FigTree-version 1.4. 3, a graphical viewer of phylogenetic trees.* 2017.
214. Ragonnet-Cronin, M., et al., *Automated analysis of phylogenetic clusters.* BMC bioinformatics, 2013. **14**(1): p. 317.
215. WHO, *World Health Organisation, Global tuberculosis report.* Geneva, 2015.
216. WHO, *World Health Organisation, Global tuberculosis report.* Geneva, 2008.
217. WHO, *Global tuberculosis report.* Geneva, 2016.
218. Kurbatova, E.V., et al., *Rifampicin-resistant Mycobacterium tuberculosis: susceptibility to isoniazid and other anti-tuberculosis drugs.* Int J Tuberc Lung Dis, 2012. **16**(3): p. 355-7.
219. Smith, S.E., et al., *Global isoniazid resistance patterns in rifampin-resistant and rifampin-susceptible tuberculosis.* Int J Tuberc Lung Dis, 2012. **16**(2): p. 203-5.
220. Moher, D., et al., *Preferred reporting items for systematic reviews and meta-analyses: the PRISMA statement.* PLoS Med, 2009. **6**(7): p. e1000097.
221. UNAIDS, *Joint United Nations Programme on HIV/AIDS.* https://www.unaids.org/en/regionscountries/countries.
222. Dramowski, A., et al., *Rifampicin-monoresistant Mycobacterium tuberculosis disease among children in Cape Town, South Africa.* Int J Tuberc Lung Dis, 2012. **16**(1): p. 76-81.
223. Menzies, H.J., et al., *Increase in anti-tuberculosis drug resistance in Botswana: results from the fourth National Drug Resistance Survey.* International Journal of Tuberculosis and Lung Disease, 2014. **18**(9): p. 1026-1033.
224. Mukinda, F.K., et al., *Rise in rifampicin-monoresistant tuberculosis in Western Cape, South Africa.* Int J Tuberc Lung Dis, 2012. **16**(2): p. 196-202.
225. Seddon, J.A., et al., *The evolving epidemic of drug-resistant tuberculosis among children in Cape Town, South Africa.* The International Journal of Tuberculosis and Lung Disease, 2012. **16**(7): p. 928-933.
226. van Halsema, C.L., et al., *Trends in drug-resistant tuberculosis in a gold-mining workforce in South Africa, 2002-2008.* Int J Tuberc Lung Dis, 2012. **16**(7): p. 967-73.
227. He, X.C., et al., *Epidemiological Trends of Drug-Resistant Tuberculosis in China From 2007 to 2014: A Retrospective Study.* Medicine (Baltimore), 2016. **95**(15): p. e3336.
228. Kruijshaar, M.E., et al., *Increasing antituberculosis drug resistance in the United Kingdom: analysis of National Surveillance Data.* Bmj, 2008. **336**(7655): p. 1231-4.
229. Lan, Y., et al., *Drug resistance profiles and trends in drug-resistant tuberculosis at a major hospital in Guizhou Province of China.* Infect Drug Resist, 2019. **12**: p. 211-219.

230. Prach, L.M., et al., *Rifampin monoresistant tuberculosis and HIV comorbidity in California, 1993-2008: a retrospective cohort study.* Aids, 2013. **27**(16): p. 2615-22.
231. Tao, N.N., et al., *Trends and characteristics of drug-resistant tuberculosis in rural Shandong, China.* Int J Infect Dis, 2017. **65**: p. 8-14.
232. Wang, P.D. and R.S. Lin, *Drug-resistant tuberculosis in Taipei, 1996-1999.* Am J Infect Control, 2001. **29**(1): p. 41-7.
233. Ridzon, R., et al., *Risk factors for rifampin mono-resistant tuberculosis.* Am J Respir Crit Care Med, 1998. **157**(6 Pt 1): p. 1881-4.
234. Sheen, P., et al., *Genetic diversity of Mycobacterium tuberculosis in Peru and exploration of phylogenetic associations with drug resistance.* PLoS One, 2013. **8**(6): p. e65873.
235. Velayati, A.A., et al., *High prevelance of rifampin-monoresistant tuberculosis: a retrospective analysis among Iranian pulmonary tuberculosis patients.* Am J Trop Med Hyg, 2014. **90**(1): p. 99-105.
236. LoBue, P.A. and K.S. Moser, *Isoniazid- and rifampin-resistant tuberculosis in San Diego County, California, United States, 1993-2002.* Int J Tuberc Lung Dis, 2005. **9**(5): p. 501-6.
237. Moore, M., et al., *Trends in drug-resistant tuberculosis in the United States, 1993-1996.* Jama, 1997. **278**(10): p. 833-7.
238. Munsiff, S.S., et al., *Rifampin-Monoresistant Tuberculosis in New York City, 1993–1994.* Clinical Infectious Diseases, 1997. **25**(6): p. 1465-1467.
239. Robert, J., et al., *Surveillance of Mycobacterium tuberculosis drug resistance in France, 1995–1997.* The International Journal of Tuberculosis and Lung Disease, 2000. **4**(7): p. 665-672.
240. Sandman, L., et al., *Risk factors for rifampin-monoresistant tuberculosis: A case-control study.* Am J Respir Crit Care Med, 1999. **159**(2): p. 468-72.
241. Vernon, A., et al., *Acquired rifamycin monoresistance in patients with HIV-related tuberculosis treated with once-weekly rifapentine and isoniazid.* The Lancet;Tuberculosis Trials Consortium, 1999. **353**(9167): p. 1843-1847.
242. Villegas, L., et al., *Prevalence, Risk Factors, and Treatment Outcomes of Isoniazid- and Rifampicin-Mono-Resistant Pulmonary Tuberculosis in Lima, Peru.* PLoS One, 2016. **11**(4): p. e0152933.
243. Nédélec, Y., et al., *Genetic ancestry and natural selection drive population differences in immune responses to pathogens.* Cell, 2016. **167**(3): p. 657-669. e21.
244. Moller, M., et al., *Genetic resistance to Mycobacterium tuberculosis infection and disease.* Frontiers in immunology, 2018. **9**: p. 2219.
245. Nikolayevsky, V., et al., *Detection of mutations associated with isoniazid and rifampin resistance in Mycobacterium tuberculosis isolates from Samara Region, Russian Federation.* Journal of clinical microbiology, 2004. **42**(10): p. 4498-4502.
246. Ahmad, S., E. Mokaddas, and E. Fares, *Characterization of rpoB mutations in rifampin-resistant clinical Mycobacterium tuberculosis isolates from Kuwait and Dubai.* Diagnostic microbiology and infectious disease, 2002. **44**(3): p. 245-252.
247. Jou, R., et al., *Genetic diversity of multidrug-resistant Mycobacterium tuberculosis isolates and identification of 11 novel rpoB alleles in Taiwan.* Journal of clinical microbiology, 2005. **43**(3): p. 1390-1394.
248. Suchindran, S., E.S. Brouwer, and A. Van Rie, *Is HIV infection a risk factor for multi-drug resistant tuberculosis? A systematic review.* PloS one, 2009. **4**(5).
249. Mesfin, Y.M., et al., *Association between HIV/AIDS and multi-drug resistance tuberculosis: a systematic review and meta-analysis.* PloS one, 2014. **9**(1).
250. Narang, P.K., et al., *Fluconazole and enhanced effect of rifabutin prophylaxis.* New England Journal of Medicine, 1994. **330**(18): p. 1316-1317.
251. Malhotra, S., et al., *A mutation in Mycobacterium tuberculosis rpoB gene confers rifampin resistance in three HIV-TB cases.* Tuberculosis, 2010. **90**(2): p. 152-157.

252. March, F., et al., *Acquired drug resistance in Mycobacterium tuberculosis isolates recovered from compliant patients with human immunodeficiency virus-associated tuberculosis.* Clinical Infectious Diseases, 1997. **25**(5): p. 1044-1047.
253. Peloquin, C.A., et al., *Low antituberculosis drug concentrations in patients with AIDS.* Annals of Pharmacotherapy, 1996. **30**(9): p. 919-925.
254. Selwyn, P.A., et al., *A prospective study of the risk of tuberculosis among intravenous drug users with human immunodeficiency virus infection.* New England journal of medicine, 1989. **320**(9): p. 545-550.
255. Faustini, A., A.J. Hall, and C.A. Perucci, *Risk factors for multidrug resistant tuberculosis in Europe: a systematic review.* Thorax, 2006. **61**(2): p. 158-163.
256. Pradipta, I.S., et al., *Risk factors of multidrug-resistant tuberculosis: A global systematic review and meta-analysis.* Journal of Infection, 2018. **77**(6): p. 469-478.
257. Law, W., et al., *Risk factors for multidrug-resistant tuberculosis in Hong Kong.* The International Journal of Tuberculosis and Lung Disease, 2008. **12**(9): p. 1065-1070.
258. Storla, D.G., S. Yimer, and G.A. Bjune, *A systematic review of delay in the diagnosis and treatment of tuberculosis.* BMC public health, 2008. **8**(1): p. 15.
259. Hirsch-Moverman, Y., et al., *Predictors of latent tuberculosis infection treatment completion in the United States: an inner city experience.* The International Journal of Tuberculosis and Lung Disease, 2010. **14**(9): p. 1104-1111.
260. Horsburgh Jr, C.R., et al., *Latent TB infection treatment acceptance and completion in the United States and Canada.* Chest, 2010. **137**(2): p. 401-409.
261. Pablos-Méndez, A., et al., *Nonadherence in tuberculosis treatment: predictors and consequences in New York City.* The American journal of medicine, 1997. **102**(2): p. 164-170.
262. Sharling, L., et al., *Rifampin-resistant Tuberculosis in the United States, 1998–2014.* Clinical Infectious Diseases, 2019.
263. Daskapan, A., et al., *A systematic review on the effect of HIV infection on the pharmacokinetics of first-line tuberculosis drugs.* Clinical pharmacokinetics, 2019. **58**(6): p. 747-766.
264. Peloquin, C., et al., *Pharmacokinetic evidence from the HIRIF trial to support increased doses of rifampin for tuberculosis.* Antimicrobial agents and chemotherapy, 2017. **61**(8).
265. Sekaggya-Wiltshire, C., et al., *Delayed Sputum Culture Conversion in Tuberculosis–Human Immunodeficiency Virus–Coinfected Patients With Low Isoniazid and Rifampicin Concentrations.* Clinical Infectious Diseases, 2018. **67**(5): p. 708-716.
266. Cox, H., et al., *Drug-resistant tuberculosis in South Africa: history, progress and opportunities for achieving universal access to diagnosis and effective treatment.* South African Health Review, 2017. **2017**(1): p. 157-167.
267. Mitchison, D. and A. Nunn, *Influence of initial drug resistance on the response to short-course chemotherapy of pulmonary tuberculosis.* American Review of Respiratory Disease, 1986. **133**(3): p. 423-430.
268. Althomsons, S. and J. Cegielski, *Impact of second-line drug resistance on tuberculosis treatment outcomes in the United States: MDR-TB is bad enough.* The International journal of tuberculosis and lung disease, 2012. **16**(10): p. 1331-1334.
269. Meyssonnier, V., et al., *Rifampicin mono-resistant tuberculosis in France: a 2005-2010 retrospective cohort analysis.* BMC Infect Dis, 2014. **14**: p. 18.
270. Seung, K.J., et al., *The effect of initial drug resistance on treatment response and acquired drug resistance during standardized short-course chemotherapy for tuberculosis.* Clinical infectious diseases, 2004. **39**(9): p. 1321-1328.
271. Zetola, N.M., et al., *Mixed Mycobacterium tuberculosis complex infections and false-negative results for rifampin resistance by GeneXpert MTB/RIF are associated with poor clinical outcomes.* Journal of clinical microbiology, 2014. **52**(7): p. 2422-2429.

272. McIvor, A., H. Koornhof, and B.D. Kana, *Relapse, re-infection and mixed infections in tuberculosis disease.* Pathogens and disease, 2017. **75**(3).
273. Williamson, D.A., et al., *An evaluation of the Xpert MTB/RIF assay and detection of false-positive rifampicin resistance in Mycobacterium tuberculosis.* Diagnostic microbiology and infectious disease, 2012. **74**(2): p. 207-209.
274. Folkvardsen, D.B., et al., *Rifampin heteroresistance in Mycobacterium tuberculosis cultures as detected by phenotypic and genotypic drug susceptibility test methods.* Journal of clinical microbiology, 2013. **51**(12): p. 4220-4222.
275. Zhang, Z., et al., *Comparison of Different Drug Susceptibility Test Methods To Detect Rifampin Heteroresistance in Mycobacterium tuberculosis.* Antimicrobial Agents and Chemotherapy, 2014. **58**(9): p. 5632-5635.
276. Kumar, P., et al., *High degree of multi-drug resistance and hetero-resistance in pulmonary TB patients from Punjab state of India.* Tuberculosis (Edinb), 2014. **94**(1): p. 73-80.
277. Zheng, C., et al., *Mixed Infections and Rifampin Heteroresistance among Mycobacterium tuberculosis Clinical Isolates.* Journal of Clinical Microbiology, 2015. **53**(7): p. 2138-2147.
278. Tang, K., et al., *Characterization of rifampin-resistant isolates of Mycobacterium tuberculosis from Sichuan in China.* Tuberculosis (Edinb), 2013. **93**(1): p. 89-95.
279. Liu, Q., et al., *Within patient microevolution of Mycobacterium tuberculosis correlates with heterogeneous responses to treatment.* Scientific Reports, 2015. **5**.
280. Shamputa, I.C., et al., *Mixed infection and clonal representativeness of a single sputum sample in tuberculosis patients from a penitentiary hospital in Georgia.* Respir Res, 2006. **7**: p. 99.
281. Doyle, R.M., et al., *Direct whole-genome sequencing of sputum accurately identifies drug-resistant Mycobacterium tuberculosis faster than MGIT culture sequencing.* Journal of clinical microbiology, 2018. **56**(8): p. e00666-18.
282. Metcalfe, J.Z., et al., *Mycobacterium tuberculosis subculture results in loss of potentially clinically relevant heteroresistance.* Antimicrobial agents and chemotherapy, 2017. **61**(11): p. e00888-17.
283. Goymer, P., *Synonymous mutations break their silence.* Nature Reviews Genetics, 2007. **8**(2): p. 92-92.
284. McCarthy, C., A. Carrea, and L. Diambra, *Bicodon bias can determine the role of synonymous SNPs in human diseases.* BMC genomics, 2017. **18**(1): p. 1-11.
285. Hofmann-Thiel, S., et al., *How should discordance between molecular and growth-based assays for rifampicin resistance be investigated?* The international journal of tuberculosis and lung disease, 2017. **21**(7): p. 721-726.
286. Mokaddas, E., et al., *Discordance between Xpert MTB/RIF assay and Bactec MGIT 960 culture system for detection of rifampin-resistant Mycobacterium tuberculosis isolates in a country with a low tuberculosis (TB) incidence.* Journal of clinical microbiology, 2015. **53**(4): p. 1351-1354.
287. Mathys, V., et al., *False-positive rifampicin resistance on Xpert® MTB/RIF caused by a silent mutation in the rpoB gene.* The International Journal of Tuberculosis and Lung Disease, 2014. **18**(10): p. 1255-1257.
288. Hirani, N., *Confirmation of silent mutations in the rpoB gene locus of M. tuberculosis isolates using pyrosequencing and phenotypic DST.* International Journal of Infectious Diseases, 2016. **45**: p. 395.
289. Alonso, M., et al., *Isolation of Mycobacterium tuberculosis strains with a silent mutation in rpoB leading to potential misassignment of resistance category.* Journal of clinical microbiology, 2011. **49**(7): p. 2688-2690.
290. Van Rie, A., et al., *False-positive rifampicin resistance on Xpert(R) MTB/RIF: case report and clinical implications.* Int J Tuberc Lung Dis, 2012. **16**(2): p. 206-8.

291. Theron, G., et al., *Evaluation of the Xpert MTB/RIF assay for the diagnosis of pulmonary tuberculosis in a high HIV prevalence setting.* Am J Respir Crit Care Med, 2011. **184**(1): p. 132-40.
292. Marlowe, E.M., et al., *Evaluation of the Cepheid Xpert MTB/RIF assay for direct detection of Mycobacterium tuberculosis complex in respiratory specimens.* J Clin Microbiol, 2011. **49**(4): p. 1621-3.
293. Ocheretina, O., et al., *False-positive rifampin resistant results with Xpert MTB/RIF version 4 assay in clinical samples with a low bacterial load.* Diagnostic microbiology and infectious disease, 2016. **85**(1): p. 53-55.
294. Ghebrekristos, Y., *Characterization of Mycobacterium tuberculosis isolates with discordant rifampicin susceptibility test results*. 2018, University of Cape Town.
295. Berhanu, R., et al. *Xpert MTB/RIF molecular probe binding characteristics associated with discordant confirmatory rifampicin resistance testing*. in *46th Union World Conference on Lung Health*. 2015.
296. Beylis, N., et al., *Characterization of Mycobacterium tuberculosis complex isolates with discordant rifampicin susceptibility test results.* Int J Tuberc Lung Dis, 2015. **46**: p. S105.
297. Hofmann-Thiel, S., et al., *Mechanisms of heteroresistance to isoniazid and rifampin of Mycobacterium tuberculosis in Tashkent, Uzbekistan.* Eur Respir J, 2009. **33**(2): p. 368-74.
298. Braden, C.R., et al., *Simultaneous infection with multiple strains of Mycobacterium tuberculosis.* Clin Infect Dis, 2001. **33**(6): p. e42-7.
299. Balganesh, M., et al., *Rv1218c, an ABC transporter of Mycobacterium tuberculosis with implications in drug discovery.* Antimicrob Agents Chemother, 2010. **54**(12): p. 5167-72.
300. Ramon-Garcia, S., et al., *Role of the Mycobacterium tuberculosis P55 efflux pump in intrinsic drug resistance, oxidative stress responses, and growth.* Antimicrob Agents Chemother, 2009. **53**(9): p. 3675-82.
301. Li, G., et al., *Study of efflux pump gene expression in rifampicin-monoresistant Mycobacterium tuberculosis clinical isolates.* J Antibiot (Tokyo), 2015. **68**(7): p. 431-5.
302. Schön, T., et al., *Rifampicin-resistant and rifabutin-susceptible Mycobacterium tuberculosis strains: a breakpoint artefact?* Journal of Antimicrobial Chemotherapy, 2013. **68**(9): p. 2074-2077.
303. Clemente, W.T., et al., *Phenotypic and genotypic characterization of drug-resistant Mycobacterium tuberculosis strains.* Diagnostic Microbiology and Infectious Disease, 2008. **62**(2): p. 199-204.
304. Williams, D.L., et al., *Characterization of rifampin-resistance in pathogenic mycobacteria.* Antimicrobial Agents and Chemotherapy, 1994. **38**(10): p. 2380-2386.
305. Bártfai, Z., et al., *Molecular Characterization of Rifampin-Resistant Isolates of Mycobacterium tuberculosis from Hungary by DNA Sequencing and the Line Probe Assay.* Journal of Clinical Microbiology, 2001. **39**(10): p. 3736-3739.
306. Gurbanova, E., et al., *Mitigation of Discordant Rifampicin-Susceptibility Results Obtained by Xpert Mycobacterium tuberculosis/Rifampicin and Mycobacterium Growth Indicator Tube.* Microb Drug Resist, 2017. **23**(8): p. 1045-1052.
307. Phelan, J., et al., *Mycobacterium tuberculosis whole genome sequencing and protein structure modelling provides insights into anti-tuberculosis drug resistance.* BMC medicine, 2016. **14**(1): p. 1-13.
308. Schleusener, V., et al., *Mycobacterium tuberculosis resistance prediction and lineage classification from genome sequencing: comparison of automated analysis tools.* Scientific reports, 2017. **7**: p. 46327.
309. Feuerriegel, S., et al., *Sequence analysis for detection of first-line drug resistance in Mycobacterium tuberculosis strains from a high-incidence setting.* BMC Microbiol, 2012. **12**: p. 90.

310. Ocheretina, O., et al., *Whole Genome Sequencing Investigation of a Tuberculosis Outbreak in Port-au-Prince, Haiti Caused by a Strain with a "Low-Level" rpoB Mutation L511P - Insights into a Mechanism of Resistance Escalation.* PLoS One, 2015. **10**(6): p. e0129207.
311. Ohno, H., et al., *Relationship between rifampin MICs for and rpoB mutations of Mycobacterium tuberculosis strains isolated in Japan.* Antimicrob Agents Chemother, 1996. **40**(4): p. 1053-6.
312. Ramaswamy, S.V., et al., *Single nucleotide polymorphisms in genes associated with isoniazid resistance in Mycobacterium tuberculosis.* Antimicrob Agents Chemother, 2003. **47**(4): p. 1241-50.
313. Yang, B., et al., *Relationship between antimycobacterial activities of rifampicin, rifabutin and KRM-1648 and rpoB mutations of Mycobacterium tuberculosis.* J Antimicrob Chemother, 1998. **42**(5): p. 621-8.
314. Campbell, E.A., et al., *Structural, functional, and genetic analysis of sorangicin inhibition of bacterial RNA polymerase.* Embo j, 2005. **24**(4): p. 674-82.
315. Jo, K.-W., et al., *Frequency and Type of Disputed rpoB Mutations in Mycobacterium tuberculosis Isolates from South Korea.* Tuberc Respir Dis, 2017. **80**(3): p. 270-276.
316. Ho, J., P. Jelfs, and V. Sintchencko, *Phenotypically occult multidrug-resistant Mycobacterium tuberculosis: dilemmas in diagnosis and treatment.* Journal of Antimicrobial Chemotherapy, 2013. **68**(12): p. 2915-2920.
317. Miotto, P., et al., *Role of Disputed Mutations in the <em>rpoB</em> Gene in Interpretation of Automated Liquid MGIT Culture Results for Rifampin Susceptibility Testing of <span class="named-content genus-species" id="named-content-1">Mycobacterium tuberculosis</span>.* Journal of Clinical Microbiology, 2018. **56**(5): p. e01599-17.
318. Domínguez, J., et al., *Clinical implications of molecular drug resistance testing for Mycobacterium tuberculosis: a TBNET/RESIST-TB consensus statement.* The International Journal of Tuberculosis and Lung Disease, 2016. **20**(1): p. 24-42.
319. Gagneux, S., et al., *The Competitive Cost of Antibiotic Resistance in <em>Mycobacterium tuberculosis</em>.* Science, 2006. **312**(5782): p. 1944.
320. Gumbo, T., *New susceptibility breakpoints for first-line antituberculosis drugs based on antimicrobial pharmacokinetic/pharmacodynamic science and population pharmacokinetic variability.* Antimicrobial agents and chemotherapy, 2010. **54**(4): p. 1484-1491.
321. Suo, J., et al., *Minimal inhibitory concentrations of isoniazid, rifampin, ethambutol, and streptomycin against Mycobacterium tuberculosis strains isolated before treatment of patients in Taiwan.* American Journal of Respiratory and Critical Care Medicine, 1988. **138**(4): p. 999-1001.
322. Turnidge, J. and D.L. Paterson, *Setting and revising antibacterial susceptibility breakpoints.* Clinical microbiology reviews, 2007. **20**(3): p. 391-408.
323. Dalhoff, A., P. Ambrose, and J. Mouton, *A long journey from minimum inhibitory concentration testing to clinically predictive breakpoints: deterministic and probabilistic approaches in deriving breakpoints.* Infection, 2009. **37**(4): p. 296-305.
324. Ramirez-Busby, S.M. and F. Valafar, *Systematic Review of Mutations in Pyrazinamidase Associated with Pyrazinamide Resistance in Mycobacterium tuberculosis Clinical Isolates.* Antimicrobial Agents and Chemotherapy, 2015. **59**(9): p. 5267-5277.
325. Whitfield, M.G., et al., *Mycobacterium tuberculosis pncA Polymorphisms That Do Not Confer Pyrazinamide Resistance at a Breakpoint Concentration of 100 Micrograms per Milliliter in MGIT.* Journal of Clinical Microbiology, 2015. **53**(11): p. 3633-3635.
326. Cynamon, M., et al., *High-dose isoniazid therapy for isoniazid-resistant murine Mycobacterium tuberculosis infection.* Antimicrobial agents and chemotherapy, 1999. **43**(12): p. 2922-2924.

327. van Ingen, J., et al., *Low-level rifampicin-resistant Mycobacterium tuberculosis strains raise a new therapeutic challenge [Short communication].* The International Journal of Tuberculosis and Lung Disease, 2011. **15**(7): p. 990-992.
328. Streicher, E., et al., *Mycobacterium tuberculosis population structure determines the outcome of genetics-based second-line drug resistance testing.* Antimicrobial agents and chemotherapy, 2012. **56**(5): p. 2420-2427.
329. Sampson, S.L., *Strength in Diversity: Hidden genetic depths of Mycobacterium tuberculosis.* Trends in microbiology, 2016. **24**(2): p. 82-84.
330. Sarathy, J.P., et al., *Prediction of drug penetration in tuberculosis lesions.* ACS infectious diseases, 2016. **2**(8): p. 552-563.
331. Gumbo, T., et al., *Concentration-dependent Mycobacterium tuberculosis killing and prevention of resistance by rifampin.* Antimicrobial agents and chemotherapy, 2007. **51**(11): p. 3781-3788.
332. Chen, H.-Y., et al., *Molecular Detection of Rifabutin-Susceptible Mycobacterium tuberculosis.* Journal of Clinical Microbiology, 2012. **50**(6): p. 2085-2088.
333. Sirgel, F.A., et al., *The rationale for using rifabutin in the treatment of MDR and XDR tuberculosis outbreaks.* PLoS One, 2013. **8**(3): p. e59414.
334. Berrada, Z.L., et al., *Rifabutin and rifampin resistance levels and associated rpoB mutations in clinical isolates of Mycobacterium tuberculosis complex.* Diagnostic microbiology and infectious disease, 2016. **85**(2): p. 177-181.
335. Chen, L., et al., *rpoB gene mutation profile in rifampicin-resistant Mycobacterium tuberculosis clinical isolates from Guizhou, one of the highest incidence rate regions in China.* Journal of Antimicrobial Chemotherapy, 2010. **65**(6): p. 1299-1301.
336. Wang, S., et al., *Molecular characterization of the rpoB gene mutations of Mycobacterium tuberculosis isolates from China* Journal of Tuberculosis Research, 2013. **01(1)**: p. 1-8.
337. Heyckendorf, J., et al., *What Is Resistance? Impact of Phenotypic versus Molecular Drug Resistance Testing on Therapy for Multi- and Extensively Drug-Resistant Tuberculosis.* Antimicrobial Agents and Chemotherapy, 2018. **62**(2): p. e01550-17.
338. Shah, N.S., et al., *Clinical Impact on Tuberculosis Treatment Outcomes of Discordance Between Molecular and Growth-Based Assays for Rifampin Resistance, California 2003–2013.* Open Forum Infectious Diseases, 2016. **3**(3).
339. Comas, I., et al., *Human T cell epitopes of Mycobacterium tuberculosis are evolutionarily hyperconserved.* Nature genetics, 2010. **42**(6): p. 498.
340. Aleksic, E., et al., *First molecular epidemiology study of Mycobacterium tuberculosis in Kiribati.* PloS one, 2013. **8**(1).
341. San, L.L., et al., *Insight into multidrug-resistant Beijing genotype Mycobacterium tuberculosis isolates in Myanmar.* International Journal of Infectious Diseases, 2018. **76**: p. 109-119.
342. Mogashoa, T., et al., *Genetic diversity of Mycobacterium tuberculosis strains circulating in Botswana.* PloS one, 2019. **14**(5).
343. Yang, C., et al., *Mycobacterium tuberculosis Beijing strains favor transmission but not drug resistance in China.* Clinical infectious diseases, 2012. **55**(9): p. 1179-1187.
344. Holt, K.E., et al., *Frequent transmission of the Mycobacterium tuberculosis Beijing lineage and positive selection for the EsxW Beijing variant in Vietnam.* Nature genetics, 2018. **50**(6): p. 849-856.
345. Bifani, P.J., et al., *Global dissemination of the Mycobacterium tuberculosis W-Beijing family strains.* Trends in microbiology, 2002. **10**(1): p. 45-52.
346. Cowley, D., et al., *Recent and rapid emergence of W-Beijing strains of Mycobacterium tuberculosis in Cape Town, South Africa.* Clinical Infectious Diseases, 2008. **47**(10): p. 1252-1259.
347. Affolabi, D., et al., *Possible outbreak of streptomycin-resistant Mycobacterium tuberculosis Beijing in Benin.* Emerging infectious diseases, 2009. **15**(7): p. 1123.

348. Van der Spuy, G., et al., *Changing Mycobacterium tuberculosis population highlights clade-specific pathogenic characteristics.* Tuberculosis, 2009. **89**(2): p. 120-125.
349. Glynn, J.R., et al., *Changes in Mycobacterium tuberculosis genotype families over 20 years in a population-based study in Northern Malawi.* PLoS One, 2010. **5**(8).
350. Gehre, F., et al., *A mycobacterial perspective on tuberculosis in West Africa: significant geographical variation of M. africanum and other M. tuberculosis complex lineages.* PLoS neglected tropical diseases, 2016. **10**(3).
351. Mbugi, E.V., et al., *Mapping of Mycobacterium tuberculosis complex genetic diversity profiles in Tanzania and other African countries.* PloS one, 2016. **11**(5).
352. Githui, W., et al., *Identification of MDR-TB Beijing/W and other Mycobacterium tuberculosis genotypes in Nairobi, Kenya.* The international journal of tuberculosis and lung disease, 2004. **8**(3): p. 352-360.
353. Rutaihwa, L.K., et al., *Multiple Introductions of the Mycobacterium tuberculosis Lineage 2 Beijing into Africa over centuries.* bioRxiv, 2018: p. 413039.
354. Andrews, J.R., et al., *Exogenous reinfection as a cause of multidrug-resistant and extensively drug-resistant tuberculosis in rural South Africa.* The Journal of infectious diseases, 2008. **198**(11): p. 1582-1589.
355. Merker, M., et al., *Evolutionary history and global spread of the Mycobacterium tuberculosis Beijing lineage.* Nature genetics, 2015. **47**(3): p. 242.
356. Tagliani, E., et al., *Culture and Next-generation sequencing-based drug susceptibility testing unveil high levels of drug-resistant-TB in Djibouti: results from the first national survey.* Scientific reports, 2017. **7**(1): p. 1-9.
357. Drobniewski, F., et al., *Drug-resistant tuberculosis, clinical virulence, and the dominance of the Beijing strain family in Russia.* Jama, 2005. **293**(22): p. 2726-31.
358. Eldholm, V., et al., *Impact of HIV co-infection on the evolution and transmission of multidrug-resistant tuberculosis.* Elife, 2016. **5**.
359. Cox, H., et al., *Delays and loss to follow-up before treatment of drug-resistant tuberculosis following implementation of Xpert MTB/RIF in South Africa: A retrospective cohort study.* PLoS Medicine, 2017. **14**(2): p. 1-19.

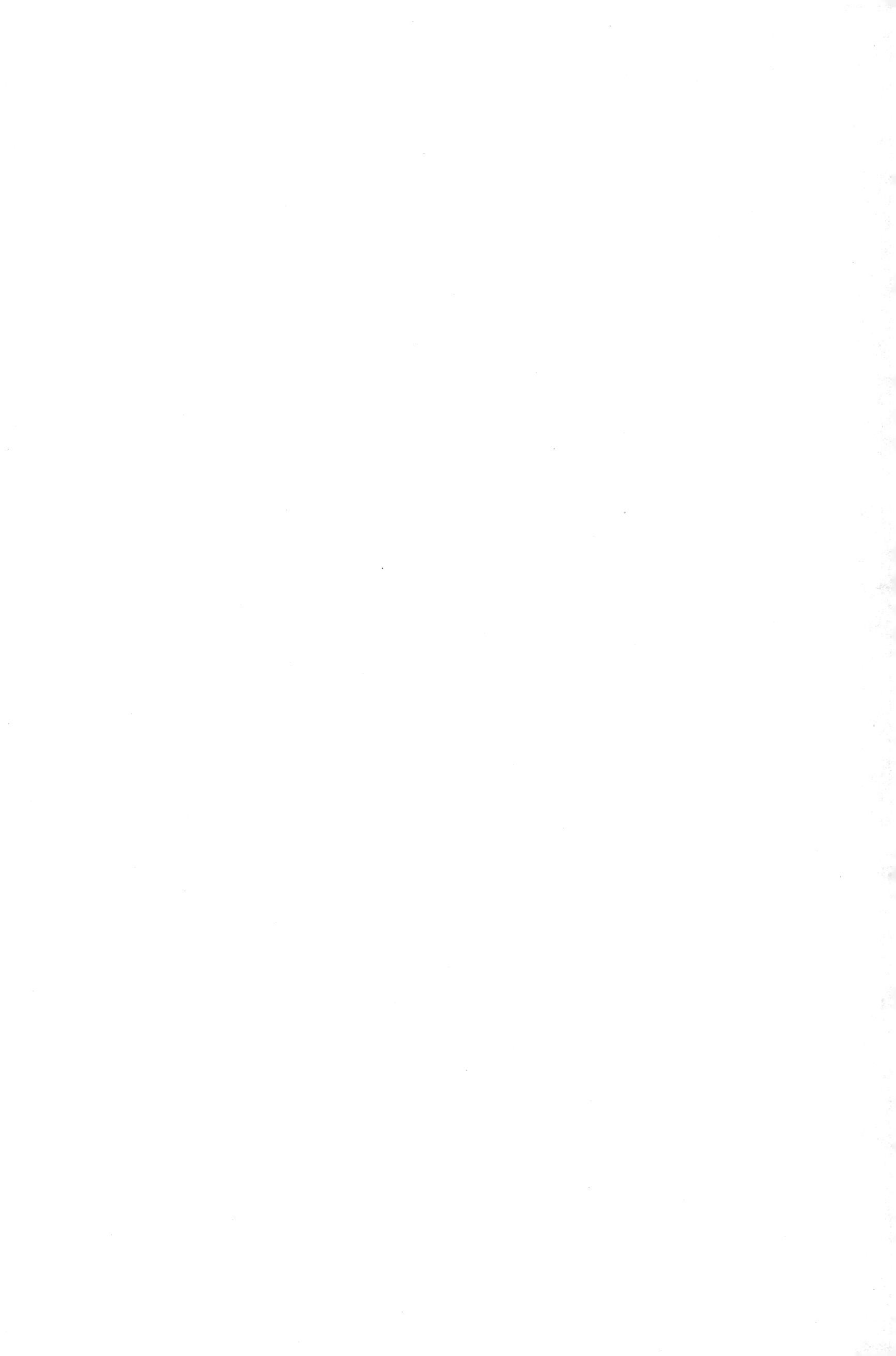

www.ingramcontent.com/pod-product-compliance
Lightning Source LLC
LaVergne TN
LVHW090935150826
845672LV00006B/1518

* 9 7 8 3 3 8 4 2 6 9 0 5 8 *